Practical Herbs 1

Henriette Kress

Front cover: The white-flowering variety of purple coneflower
(*Echinacea purpurea*).

Back cover: Rosebay willowherb (fireweed) (*Epilobium angustifolium*).

First published in Finland in 2011.

This edition published 2018 by

Aeon Books Ltd
Hilltop
Lewes BN7 3HS

British Library Cataloguing in Publication Data
A C.I.P. for this book is available from the British Library
ISBN-13: 978-1-91159-757-5

www.aeonbooks.co.uk

PREFACE

I'm an herbalist who lives and works in Finland, in northern Europe, and the herbs I've selected to write about reflect this. These 23 herbs are either abundant in Finnish woods and meadows or are easily grown in Finnish gardens.

However, these herbs have a circumboreal appeal. If you live anywhere near the temperate zone, for example, you're likely to find dandelion, stinging nettles, or horsetail growing in the wild. If you have a yard or garden, you may grow roses, calendula, and California poppy.

In addition to herbs, I cover many other topics: how to pick herbs and what to do with them once they're picked; how to make herbal oils, salves, and tinctures; which minor ailments can benefit from herbal treatment, and which medicinal herbs can also be used as food.

And, of course, how to make your own rose beads.

ACKNOWLEDGMENTS

I thank everyone who asked questions and shared their experiences with me during my lectures.

I thank my wonderful clients, who have helped me gain experience using herbs to treat a variety of disorders as they manifest in different types of people.

I thank all the herbalists and herbal hobbyists who have shared their knowledge, experiences, and tips in online forums, blogs, and websites.

I thank those who have proofread this text.

Finally, I reserve my most heartfelt thanks for my teachers, now deceased—my grandmother E. Brennecke and herbalist Michael Moore.

I wish you much joy in the world of herbs!

Henriette Kress
October 2011

A new edition, enjoy!
Henriette Kress, November 2020

TABLE OF CONTENTS

The Plants

Index

THE BASICS

—picking, drying, and preparing your herbs.

PICKING HERBS

Before you take your basket and go out picking, remember these rules.

IDENTIFICATION

Pick only the herbs you know. Learn to tell dandelion (*Taraxacum*) from coltsfoot (*Tussilago farfara*), sow thistle (*Sonchus oleraceus*), and other look-alike yellow-flowering composite plants. Learn how stinging nettle (*Urtica dioica*) differs from, say, white deadnettle (*Lamium album*), and how shepherd's purse (*Capsella bursa-pastoris*) differs from a host of pennycresses (*Thlaspi* species) and similar mustard-family plants.

Be especially careful with the umbellifers. Before you pick even one Angelica, be sure you know how to tell this beneficial species from its deadly doubles the water hemlocks (*Cicuta* species). Edible and medicinal fern-leafed umbellifers can closely resemble the deadly poison

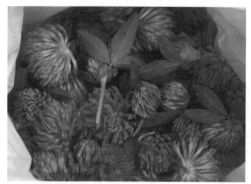

Red clover flowers in a paper bag.

hemlock (*Conium maculatum*).

Don't pick large quantities of an herb you've finally located after years of searching. Instead, pluck a twig, a flower, and a leaf, and take those home with you. Then double-check what you wanted the plant for, and which part of the plant you should gather for that purpose.

Once you've identified a plant in the wild, you'll spot it more easily in the future.

PICKING RIGHTS

In Finland and Sweden we have a law called "Every Man's Right," which permits the gathering for personal use of aboveground parts of nonwoody plants in forests and meadows. We may take only berries from woody plants, and we may not pick aboveground parts in quantities large enough to sell. We are prohibited from digging roots or taking lichens and mosses without a landowner's permission.

Learn your local laws—and always seek permission before gathering anything from private property. Be polite: take only what you need, and leave the area looking nice. Share some of your herbal products with your host, and you'll be welcome to return.

Always leave endangered and rare plants to grow and prosper.

HEALTHY PLANTS

Gather parts from only clean and healthy plants.

You need not go to extremes: leave plants with leaves eaten to a lace to recover. Also leave plants with signs of fungal diseases (powdery mildew, orange spots, and the like).

Remove any damaged leaves before using.

UNPOLLUTED AREA

When you go out to gather herbs, walk beyond the range of dust from dirt roads, or 75 feet from a paved road, 300 feet from a highway, or a half-mile from a freeway.

Avoid plants that grow near stables, in pastures, or behind outhouses. These areas host an abundance of gut bacteria—essential for our digestion but not all that healthful to ingest! And with so much fertilizer about, any plants that accumulate nitrates will certainly have done so.

Keep away from conventionally farmed fields. However, margins of organically farmed fields can be excellent picking spots. Just don't step into the crops.

Large cities and industrial areas inevitably are the most polluted, yet you'll find people cultivating gardens on their small plots even there. Check out an area's history: a factory may be long-gone, but its toxic waste will be everpresent.

PROTECT THE STANDS

If the herb species you're reaching for is the only one of its kind you see, leave it.

If it's one of a very few, leave it.

If it's a prolific grower, such as stinging nettle, dandelion, yellow dock, or willowherb, pick at most half the aboveground parts, or dig at most a fifth of the roots.

If the plant is a perennial, wait until the plant has set seed before you dig the root.

Don't be greedy. Take only as much as you need. Plan on coming back for more of the same herb for years to come, and pick accordingly.

PICKING EQUIPMENT

The best containers to pick into are lightweight yet sturdy. I quite like baskets woven from natural materials.

Bring scissors (or clippers, or a knife), gloves (thick enough to protect your hands from irritants such as nettles), and paper bags (that way you can put each species into its own bag and avoid, for example, the yarrow taking on the scent and flavor of meadowsweet).

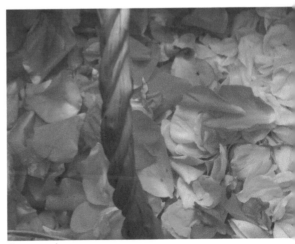

Rose petals.

HARVESTING TIME

The best time to pick flowers and leaves is when the plants are fully grown but not yet damaged by insects or diseases. (In Finland, this is mid-July.)

It's usually best to pick the flowering tops, except for plants such as willowherb (*Epilobium* species), which form seedpods that explode into room-filling fluff during drying.

Dig roots in the fall, when aboveground parts are brown and dead. If it's rainy, windy, and dreary outside, dig roots in the spring, instead: it may be just as rainy, windy, and dreary, but it feels so good to go out and dig after a long winter.

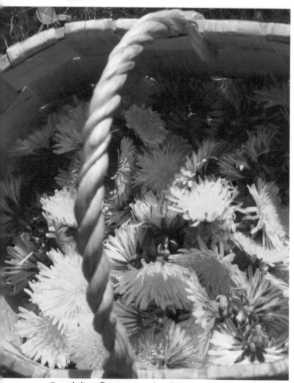

Dandelion flowers in a basket.

Take the roots of biennials such as carrot and burdock after the plant's first summer. The plump, sweet root of the first autumn becomes a stringy anchor for the flowerstalk by the second summer, and then a rotted husk after the seeds mature.

Pick seed heads when a plant's stems start to turn brown. Pick single seeds when they're mature but before they fall off on their own.

PROCESSING YOUR HARVEST

Plants spoil as easily as fungi or fish, so always clean and process your herbs the same day you pick them.

Factor this into your schedule: it can take twice as long to wash and process roots as it takes to pick them, for example.

If you clean your leafy harvest before you add it to your basket, it becomes easy to process. All it needs now is a quick check: did you miss any many-legged proteins or bird poop? Remove those, and your harvest is ready to be dried or tinctured.

The less time you spend outside gathering plants, the more time you'll spend inside cleaning them. (If I have to battle mosquitoes and horseflies, I pick fast and clean indoors!)

CLEANUP

Be considerate. Leave any area you gather from at least as tidy as it was when you arrived.

Refill the holes you dig to prevent twisted ankles later on—yours or someone else's.

Conceal discarded stems and the like under nearby foliage.

DRYING YOUR HERBS

You can preserve your herbs in a variety of ways: drying, freezing, tincturing, or making them into an oil or vinegar.

Drying is the easiest way to preserve herbs for later use. Dried well, they have almost the same color and scent as when they were fresh. There are several ways to do this.

HANGING

For whole plants, cut the plant below the lowest healthy leaves. Remove damaged, dirty, and yellowing parts. Rinse any dirt-splattered plants, and then dry them carefully between layers of cotton cloth or towels, or use a salad spinner.

Gather 10 to 15 stems and secure them tightly where the stem bundle is thickest using cotton string, twine, or even stout rubber bands. The plants will shrink as they dry, and if you bind them too loosely some may fall out. Herbs you've rinsed may still be a bit wet, so tie them instead into very small bundles of five to seven stems to keep mold from forming.

Hang your bundles in a dry place indoors out of the light.

Your herbs are dry when both the thickest and the thinnest stems break when you bend them. Now you are ready to strip the stems or cut them up for storage in glass jars with tight-fitting lids.

This method is inappropriate for plants that lose important parts as they dry. The drying flowers of German chamomile, for instance, tend to drop their yellow centers—the strongest part of the plant.

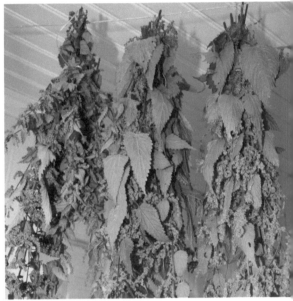

Nettles in seed, drying in bundles.

> **Tip:** *Tie a bundle of herbs to each end of a short length of twine or string. This way, rather than struggle to knot each bunch in place, you can just toss one over your drying line or rack to suspend them both.*
>
> *Pull one of the bundles down; the other will go up. This will help the bundles dry faster.*

Stripping the stems

Spread a clean cotton bed sheet on the floor. Cut down all the bundles of one herb and put them in the middle of your sheet. Put on your gloves (to protect your fingers from splinters), and strip the stems. Some parts may fly off, but most will stay on the sheet. Once you've stripped the lot, lift the sheet corners to gather in the strays, and you'll get a neat pile of herbs.

Cutting the stems

Some herb plants are best cut into 1-inch (2–3 cm) lengths. The stems of hyssop, for instance, work just as well as leaves.

You'll find storing cut stems requires more containers, though.

For example, where the cut flowering stems of hyssop takes up three quart jars, its stripped-off flowers and leaves would have needed only one.

Other drawbacks: It takes more time to cut up stems.

Your hands get tired.

Your fingers may develop blisters.

FLAT DRYING

Although it's true that the more crushed and crumbled they are, the more dried herb parts you can fit in their glass jars, leaves and flowers that are kept whole retain their constituents better.

Roots and fruit should first be scrubbed (if very dirty) or rinsed. You needn't scrub off the root bark, but do remove dead or damaged parts.

Next, cut them into quarter-inch (5 mm) slices or sticks. Long, thin roots dry more evenly if they're sliced open, even if they're very narrow.

Dry your prepared herbs on racks at temperatures no higher than 104 °F (40 °C).

Dehydrator

A dehydrator is very useful for drying roots or fruit. (Of course, it can also be used for other plant parts, and for drying fungi or meat. Scrub your dehydrator trays often!)

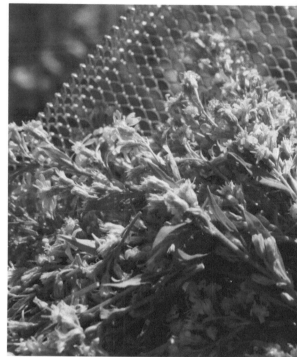

*Goldenrod (*Solidago *species) on a drying rack.*

If you're drying a strong-scented species, fill the dehydrator with just that one herb. Mixed species will acquire the scent of the strongest-smelling plants as they dry.

Load unscented or mildly scented herbs any way you prefer, as long as you can separate the different species once the parts are dry.

You can build your own dehydrator or buy one. The best have temperature settings and inbuilt timers. Make sure the factory-set minimum temperature is low enough. A dehydrator set higher than 122 °F (50 °C) will toast your herbs rather than dry them.

Oven

Many people dry plants successfully in older gas ovens using just the heat of the pilot light.

Electric ovens, however, aren't perfect for drying herbs. You may set the temperature to 122 °F (50 °C), but an older oven can well heat up to 194 °F (90 °C) overnight. By then, your herbs have burned.

Leaving the oven door open a crack doesn't help: the herbs nearest the door will stay moist enough to make the whole batch go moldy; the herbs in the middle will be nice and dry; the herbs farthest back will be burned (even if the rest of the batch is sufficiently dry, they'll still taste burned.

I thought convection ovens might solve the problem, but some types stop heating if the oven door isn't shut all the way. And convection means the oven air circulates, nevermind how damp it is.

Microwave oven

Microwaving boils the water out of the herb. Although people have told me they've gotten prime dried parsley and similar culinary herbs using their microwave oven, I won't use one to dry medicinal herbs.

Drying cabinet

If you own a drying cabinet, you can use it to dry your herbs, too—but not together with clothes! Set the temperature to a maximum of 104 °F (40 °C). Remember to leave the cabinet door open.

Wood-burning cookstove

An old-fashioned wood-burning cookstove is very good for drying herbs: fire it up at one end, and place a drying rack atop a few bricks at the other.

Sauna

If you're not using your sauna, spread your herbs on an old bed sheet there.

Drying without extra heat

Spread your cleaned herbs (don't mix species!) on an old bed sheet or a other large square of clean cotton fabric on a thick layer of newspapers out of the light in any indoor corner. If you have pets or small children, the floor will be an unsuitable surface. A tabletop or the top of a seldom-used chest freezer work well.

Your herbs will shrink in volume by half in about three days. If the summer is dry, they should be completely dry in about nine days. Changing the underlying newspapers every couple of days speeds the drying process.

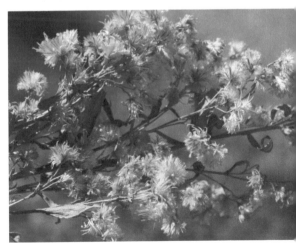

Dried flowering tops of goldenrod. The brownish-yellow fluff is a normal part of the dried herb.

STORING DRIED HERBS

If you're out of glass jars, put your herbs temporarily into paper or plastic bags. Move them to tightly lidded glass jars as soon as possible. Keep the jars in the dark: a closed cupboard at room temperature is good.

Never put moist or not-quite-dry herbs into lidded jars. They'll grow mold in no time.

Label the jar with the herb's name and the date you picked it. A month or twelve down the road you might still know the herb by appearance, scent, or taste, but do you remember the year you gathered it? It's helpful to include the location where you found the plant on the label, as well—for example, "Nettles, July 7 2021, Grandma's garden."

SHELF LIFE OF DRIED HERBS

As a rule of thumb, an herb's green parts will have lost their usefulness after a year or so, roots and bark after about two years.

But taste or sniff your herbs: *Ooh—nice, the meadowsweet keeps getting stronger in its jar. It will do for another year.* Or, *This angelica root's flavor has faded a little. It won't work anymore.* Feed it to the compost heap, or make a footbath from it.

And if you want your yarrow root to actually work for toothache, you must collect new roots every other year, or even every year. Four-year-old roots are useless.

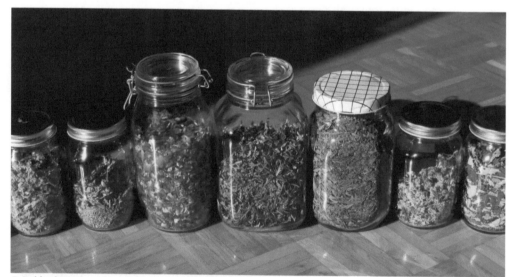

Dried herbs in jars. From left to right: meadowsweet flowers (Filipendula ulmaria), flowering tops of musk-mallow (Malva moschata), rose petals, green leaf of arborvitae (Thuja occidentalis), the leaf of rosebay willowherb (Epilobium angustifolium), yarrow flowers (Achillea species), and red raspberry leaf (Rubus idaeus).

MAKING AND USING HERBAL TEAS

There are three basic ways to make herbal teas:
- pour boiling water on the fresh or dried herb and let steep (infusion);
- bring the herb parts to a boil in water, then let simmer or steep (decoction);
- steep the herb in cold water (maceration or cold infusion, nourishing infusion).

Make one day's worth of tea at a time. Bacteria can grow in the refrigerator, too.

If you plan on using your herbal tea for a cough, add some sugar, honey, or the like: sugar increases mucus production.

Don't sweeten teas you use for digestive problems. The digestion of sugar will disrupt an herb's activity.

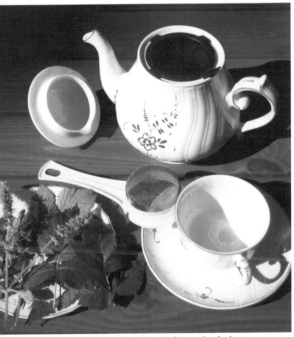

Everything you need to make an herbal tea.

HOW TO MAKE AN INFUSION

Infusions are generally made from the soft parts of herbs—flowers, tops, and leaves.

For each cup, use 1 or 2 teaspoons of dried herb, or 2 to 4 teaspoons fresh, with 1 cup (250 ml) boiling water. Pour boiling water over the herb, steep 5 to 10 minutes, strain, and drink.

You can safely drink up to five cups a day of the milder herbs.

HOW TO MAKE A DECOCTION

Decoctions are usually made from the harder herbs or parts of herbs, such as bark, lichen, hard fruit, and larger seeds.

For each cup, add 1 or 2 teaspoons dried herb, or 2 to 4 teaspoons fresh herb to 1 cup (250 ml) cold water in a pan, bring to a boil, and simmer for 5 to 10 minutes. Remove the pan from the heat, let steep 5 to 10 minutes more, strain, and drink.

HOW TO MAKE A MACERATION

Maceration, also called cold infusion, is suited to any herbal part. I recommend against macerating herbs that are high in tannins, however. Your finished tea will be quite bitter.

For each cup, add 1 or 2 teaspoons dried herb, or 2-4 teaspoons fresh, to 1 cup (250 ml) cold water in a suitable container. Let stand overnight in your refrigerator. In the morning, strain out the herb, and drink. You may also bring the cold maceration to a boil before straining.

Mucilaginous herbs such as mallows and mullein are perfect for macerations.

NICE HERBS FOR TEA BLENDS

Use mild herbs such as willowherb or cinquefoil leaves as a base for your tea. Mallows (leaf, flower, or root) give body to any tea you add them to.

Choose an herb to give your tea its dominant flavor. For instance:

- Minty: peppermint, Japanese mint, showy calamint, mountain mints
- Lemony: lemon balm, lemon verbena, lemon catmint, Moldavian balm, roselle, lemon grass, lemon thyme
- Anise overtones: sweet chervil, anise hyssop, young leaves of goutweed, aniseed, fennel seeds
- Herbal: basil, thyme, hyssop, sweet marjoram, tarragon, sage
- Hot: bee balms, ginger, and, if picked during a hot summer, basil and savory
- Berry: leaves of black currant, red raspberry, strawberry, or bilberry
- Sweet: licorice, stevia
- Mineral: nettles, horsetail, lady's mantle, sunflower leaf, green oats
- Interesting: give sweet flag (*Acorus calamus*) a twirl in your cuppa
- Surprising: try pineapple sage or scented geranium leaves. They taste like their scent!

Add something to complement the dominant note. For example:

- a few rose petals give interest to the spices
- just a hint of mint adds that little extra to the mineral herbs
- a little bitter is nice in lemony tea combinations

This sampling is far from complete.

FERMENTING

Fermenting can give a different, sometimes finer, aroma to herbs. "Black tea," for example, is fermented green tea.

Start by crushing the fresh leaf to bring its juices to the surface. Leave the bruised parts somewhere warm overnight. Finally, dry your now-darkened herbs.

To crush fresh herbs for fermenting, I have tried every trick in the book:

- placing herbs in a plastic bag, removing all the air from it, and then pressing them firmly under a rolling pin;
- stomping on the bagged herbs with wooden clogs;
- crushing the leaves one by one in the diligent hands of many friends;
- recruiting friends to roll "cigars" from up to 10 leaves at a time, and then cutting the cigars into small pieces.

I find these methods so heavy on the work and light on the fun that I'd rather not bother.

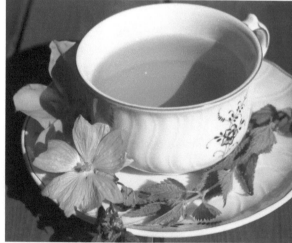

A cup of herbal tea made with nettles, mallow, and a little rose.

If you own a pasta maker, however, you have it made. Set the flat rolls as close together as possible, put the crank in place, and crank your herb leaves through, one by one or a few at a time. The machine crushes leaves nicely and makes quick work of a basketful.

And it gets better: if you then crank the leaves through the thinnest "spaghetti" part of the machine, they'll be all sliced up!

Put the crushed herb in a glass jar with a loosened lid. Set the jar in a warm spot—say, 122 °F (50 °C)—overnight. The top of a large dehydrator works nicely.

In the morning, spread the fermented material to dry on a cloth or baking parchment, or in dehydrator trays.

Finally, store your bone-dry tea leaves in an airtight jar and label (example: "Red raspberry leaf, fermented, July 2021").

Herbs that lend themselves to fermenting include rowan leaf, rosebay willowherb leaf, and the leaves of various brambles such as blackberry, stone bramble or arctic blackberry.

AN HERBAL BATH

  2–3 handfuls dried herbs
  2 quarts (liters) water

Bring the water to a boil, add the herbs, steep for 10 to 20 minutes, and strain.

Pour the strained liquid into your almost-ready bath and adjust the temperature.

Enjoy your bath for 20 to 30 minutes.

A FOOTBATH

Herbs well-suited for footbaths include stinging nettles, willowherb, meadowsweet, and horsetail.

  1–2 quarts (liters) fresh herbs
  2 quarts (liters) water

Twist the herbs into 2–4-inch (5–10 cm) lengths, put them in a pan, and add water. Bring to a boil, and then simmer for 10 to 20 minutes.

To enjoy your footbath outdoors, pour your water-and-herbs into a basin. Add a few flowers for decoration.

Indoors, strain the herbs out first.

Either way, add cold water until the bath is hot but not scalding. Take off your shoes and socks, pull up your trouser legs, sit down with your feet in the water, and wiggle your toes for 10 to 20 minutes. Lovely!

Tip: *Add nettles first to the boiling water and allow them to wilt thoroughly.*

Otherwise, they'll still sting—refreshing, perhaps, but not all that comfortable.

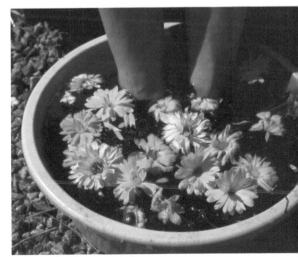

A footbath with calendula flowers.

HERBAL OILS

Herbal oils are a great way to get herbs onto your skin.

WHICH OIL SHOULD I USE?

The best oils are light (for rapid absorption), contain a lot of vitamin E (to keep them fresh longer), are cold-pressed (so that if they do go rancid you'll notice it from the smell), and are from organically grown plants (no pesticide residues).

It's also good if the oil is odorless or pleasantly scented.

Herb books usually tell you to use olive oil because it contains so much vitamin E, but almost all cold-pressed oils contain large amounts of that vitamin: olive oil, sesame seed oil, safflower oil, rapeseed (canola) oil and the like.

If you're like me and don't like olive oil, try another oil. Keep it in the fridge for added shelf life.

- Extra-virgin olive oil is a traditionally used, strong-scented oil.

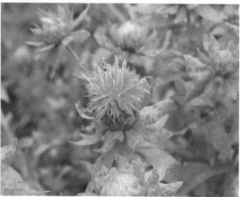

Safflower in bloom. The oil is pressed from its seeds.

- Safflower oil is light and odorless.
- Sesame seed oil absorbs quickly into the skin and has a pleasant scent. (But reserve the roasted, dark sesame seed cooking oil for your wok!)
- Almond and walnut oils are exquisite—light, and expensive—and people can be allergic to them. They also go rancid quickly.
- Rapeseed (canola) oil is an easy choice in Finland, as it's found in all grocery stores. Make sure the brand you select doesn't smell too strongly. If you use it in your salves, you'll need to use additional beeswax.

WHICH HERB SHOULD I USE?

- Calendula flowers soothe the skin and help heal wounds. I include them in almost all my salves.
- Plantain (*Plantago*) leaf is another good wound healer. The species grows almost everywhere, but picking it in the wild can be time-consuming.
- Flowering tops of St. John's wort (*Hypericum* species) make an excellent oil for treating trauma damage—sprains, bruises, contusions—as well as some joint problems. It's also good for treating wounds and for soothing nerves—both physiological and emotional. (The oil of St. John's wort smells of olive oil no matter what you infuse it in.)
- Arborvitae (*Thuja* species), cypress, and cedar green parts help kill fungi on the skin. They're not strong enough to treat nail fungi, however.
- Goldenrod relieves most muscle aches. Try it for pains nothing else has touched. Give the oil a try for itches and swellings, too.

- Meadowsweet (*Filipendula ulmaria*) flowers and green parts treat a variety of aches and pains.
- Balsam poplar (*Populus balsamifera*) leaf buds are even stronger than meadowsweet, but picking them can be messy: everything you've touched during the harvest is now covered in a sticky resin.
- True mints cool and refresh. Massaged into temples, the infused oil can even help with headaches. Peppermint variety "Mitcham" (sometimes classified *Mentha piperita* var. *rubra*) which contains a lot of menthol, is ideal for this purpose.
  A mint salve requires extra beeswax to make it solidify.
- Rose and lavender flowers are scented and calming. They help heal wounds and soothe inflamed skin. Rose-scented oils and salves require a scentless oil and strongly scented petals. The more robust lavender can overpower the scent of sesame oil but not rapeseed (canola) oil.
- Horse chestnut (*Aesculus hippo-castanum*) leaf, bark, and sliced-up green seed (and pod) help strengthen capillaries. Use the infused oil externally to treat rosacea and to tighten up varicose veins, hemorrhoids, and bags under the eyes.
- Fresh dandelion flowers make a good oil for relaxing tense muscles, especially if they were tense because of emotions—frustration, anger, or irritation. Try it for a stress-tensed neck, too!
- Garden cucumber, leaves of chickweed (*Stellaria media*), and *Impatiens* species make an oil that calms itches and inflamed skin.
- Mullein (*Verbascum* species) flowers and leaf help fight inflammations.
  I cut the flower stalk and use it all—flower buds, flowers, seedpods—and even the stalk, if it's slender enough. The infused

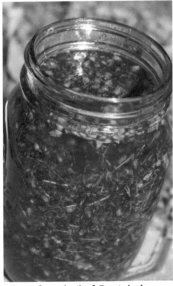

I haven't used the leave-your-herbal-oil-on-the-windowsill-for-weeks method for years. That way, my herbal oil won't go rancid before I even strain it, nor will any herb parts above the oil grow mold.

The infused oil of St. John's wort is made from fresh flowering tops.The dried herb won't color the oil red.

oil is excellent for earaches: place a few drops in the achy ear (two or three drops for an adult, one drop for a child), or rub a few drops behind it.
Mullein-infused oil and salve are also good for tense muscles and tendonitis. (If you have the latter, by the way, please get more magnesium into your daily diet, either from magnesium-rich food or a supplement.)

Never use infused oils internally unless they are made from dried herbs. (See page 20).

DRIED OR FRESH?

I use dried herbs for infused oils almost exclusively. That way, I needn't wait for the oil to clear and moisture to settle to the bottom of the jar—which can take from four to seven days. An oil made from fresh frozen herb can take up to two weeks to clear.

I do use use fresh plants when I make infused oil of St. John's wort, however; the dried herb won't give you a nice red oil.

My infused oils of chickweed, cucumber, and our local Impatiens species are also made from fresh herbs: their cooling and skin-calming effects are due to juices that are lost in drying.

HOW TO MAKE HERBAL OILS

Place your plant material in the oil you've chosen (see the foregoing section, "Which oil should I use?"), steep, and then strain out the material when it's done.

Traditionally, one jams herbs into a jar, covers them with oil, and leaves them on a sunny windowsill for several weeks. But I prefer to infuse most of my herbal oils in a water bath (bain-marie or double boiler).

A fast oil in a water bath

2 cups (500 ml) oil
fresh or dried herbs

A Pyrex or enameled double-boiler is ideal for this. In the absence of a double-boiler, pour water into a saucepan and suspend a bowl over the water so its sides don't

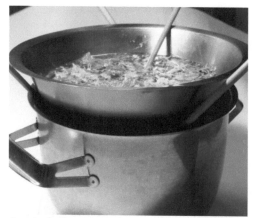

A water bath—water in the pan, calendula and oil in the bowl.

touch the pan itself. Three untreated bamboo chopsticks work well for this.

Pour oil into the bowl. Cut your fresh herbs into 1-inch lengths (2–3 cm), or crush your dried herb. Add as much herb as possible to the oil: don't add so much that you end up with heaps of dried herb on top of the oil, but don't add so little that you have herbless areas in the oil, either. If your bowl is small enough, and you infuse enough herbs and oil, a knife stood in the bowl should stay upright for a while.

Bring the water to a boil, and then lower the heat to keep it at a simmer. Add water as needed to keep the pan from boiling dry.

Leave your oil on your water bath between 90 minutes and two hours. Take care the oil doesn't boil or smoke: you're making an infused herb oil, not fried herbs.

Lift the bowl off the pan and let the oil cool for about 30 minutes. Then wipe the sides and the rim of the bowl and strain the oil into another clean vessel.

If you used dried herbs, your oil is now done. Pour it into a bottle, cap tightly, and add a label (example: "Herbal oil, sesame seed oil, dried meadowsweet, and calendula, August 2021").

If you used fresh herbs, now you must let the water separate from the oil. Pour the strained oil into a wide-mouthed jar and let it settle in a corner (sunny for St. John's wort; shady for other herbs) for four to seven days (up to two weeks, if you used fresh frozen herbs)—that is, until the oil clears. Pour the oil carefully off the bottom muck, bottle, and label (example: "Herbal oil, safflower oil, fresh St. John's wort, July 2021").

Tips for a bain-marie

In a bain-marie, water-bath, or double-boiler, water heats in one vessel under another suspended above it.

To improvise your own bain-marie, simply suspend a bowl above a saucepan of boiling water. Experience has taught me that the form and size of the bowl are important:

• The bowl's diameter must be greater than the pan's. Otherwise the bowl can easily tip on its side in the boiling water. Rescuing the bowl with your fingers is painful! And with a utensil it's cumbersome.

• A round bowl can again tip over easily, and likewise will be difficult to rescue.

STRAINING YOUR OIL

To strain the oil you've made from dried or fresh plant parts, spread a square of clean cheesecloth about 16 by 16 inches (40 by 40 cm) over a clean, dry bowl so that its corners lie outside the bowl's opening. You should have enough room for the oil-and-herb mess to fit in the middle of the cloth. Pour the mixture into the cloth.

Gathering the corners of the cloth in one hand, get a good grip on the herbs with the other and wring as much liquid from it as you can. When you've extracted most of the oil this way, fold over the dry part of the cloth and wring hard again with both hands.

To strain oil from powdered herbs, pour it into a large coffee filter in a sieve suspended over a dry, clean bowl, and let it drip through overnight. Suspend the sieve high enough to keep it from touching the oil as it accumulates in the bowl.

PROBLEMS WITH HERBAL OILS

What can go wrong when you make an infused herbal oil?

• Your oil can rot. This happens all too often if you use fresh herbs and the "jar on a windowsill" method. The smell is absolutely disgusting.

• Your herb can grow mold. When you jam herbs into a glass jar and cover the herbs with oil, you'll always have the odd leaf, stem or flower above the oil. If you don't stir your oil often enough they'll grow mold in a matter of days.

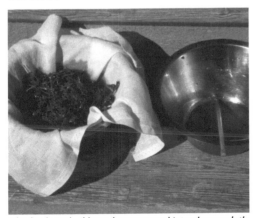

The herb and oil have been poured into cheesecloth.

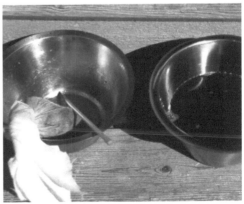

The oil is strained.

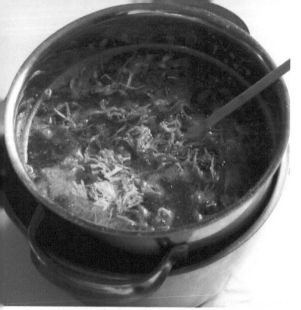

A water bath: a smaller pan in a larger one. The herbs are calendula and rose.

- Your oil may escape from its jar. If you infuse fresh herbs in oil in a glass jar, you can find an astonishing amount of oil outside the jar each morning. A saucer won't catch it all; a deep plate or ceramic or Pyrex pie plate will. Pour the escaped oil back into the jar.
- The oil goes rancid. You can't stop it but you can slow it:
  —Use Vitamin E as an antioxidant. Add straight vitamin E oil, 0.34 fluid ounces (10 ml) per quart (liter) of oil. Note that vitamin E is messy.
  —Use a recently pressed oil, which won't go rancid for at least a year.
  —Refrigerate your oils during hot summer months.
- You find a gelatinous mass floating in your oil. If you make an infused oil from fresh herb parts, you may end up with a translucent gel in your bottle of oil no matter how closely you followed instructions. Never fear. The oil proteins have simply reacted with one or another herb constituent. If you heat the oil, the gel will dissolve. You may use the oil with no problem.

BACTERIA IN OILS

Anaerobic bacteria in oil pose no danger when used externally. But if you want to ingest your oil, please consider the following.

Oil creates an oxygen-free environment. Fresh herb parts contain water. Put an oxygen-free environment together with water and you've made an excellent breeding ground for anaerobic bacteria.

The most dangerous of these bacteria is *Clostridium botulinum*, which produces the botulism toxin. This poison is without scent, color, or taste, and this bacterium won't make jar lids bulge.

Botulism toxin can kill or paralyze in extremely small amounts. Because the botulinum bacterium is commonly found in soil, it can attach itself to plant surfaces, especially those dug out of the ground, such as garlic. Spores of this bacterium can even be found in raw honey. The bacteria and spores aren't toxic in themselves, but the live bacterium exudes the botulism toxin.

Adults and children over a year old generally have sufficient stomach acid to kill the bacteria, but stomach acid can't affect any toxin the bugs already have produced. This is why you must make your herbal oils inhospitable to anaerobic bacteria.

For example:

- Add unadulterated salt. If the salinity of your oil is over 7 percent, the spores won't develop into bacteria, and there will be no toxin in the finished product.
- Use only dried herbs in your herbal oils. Nothing can grow without water, not even the botulinum bacterium.

• Make sure your oil is sufficiently acidic. If you lower the pH to below 4.5, the spores won't develop into bacteria. Add too much vinegar to your oil, though, and it will taste of vinegar.

• Use up your oil within three days, and keep it refrigerated. The spores won't have time enough to develop into bacteria.

None of these tricks will destroy botulism toxin once it's been produced. To destroy the spores or the bacteria, you must keep all the oil at 176 to 212 °F (80 to 100 °C) for ten minutes. You must maintain the temperature evenly for 30 minutes to render the toxin harmless.

Unfortunately, after such treatment your oil will go rancid much faster. And if you had herbs in your oil during the heating, now they're probably both boiled and fried.

THE DIFFERENCE BETWEEN INFUSED AND ESSENTIAL OILS

Volatile, ethereal, or essential oils are single active constituents—or, more precisely, groupings of similar single constituents—concentrates distilled or chemically extracted from a large amount of crude herbs. You will get at most a pint (500 ml) of essential oil from 220 pounds (100 kg) of fresh lavender buds.

An essential oil won't leave a greasy stain on paper. Because it's volatile, it will evaporate, leaving behind its scent and a little color.

Aromatherapists work with scent using essential oils that have been diluted in fatty oils (food oils).

Herbalists apply infused herbal oils (herbs in fatty or food oils) and the salves made from them directly to the skin.

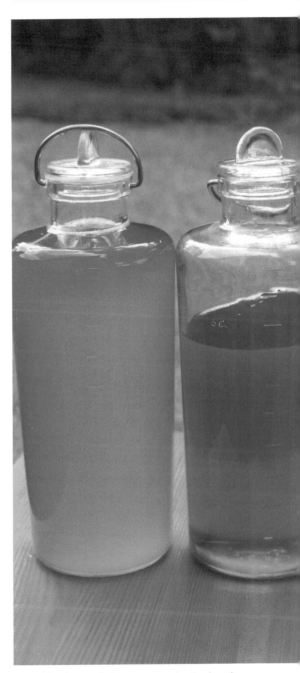

Oils of fresh St. John's wort—one cloudy, the other cleared.

21

HERBAL SALVES

Salves are made by by melting beeswax in a strained infused herbal oil. They aren't as messy as oils, and you will use less of a salve than you would of the same oil.

A BASIC HERBAL SALVE

> 3 cups (750 ml) herbal oil (page 18)
> 4 ounces (100 g) beeswax

Heat the oil in a bain-marie or double-boiler. If your beeswax is in thin sheets (1–2 mm), tear it into strips and add to the heated oil. If you have beeswax buttons, add them whole.

Keep the water of your bain-marie at a full boil, or your beeswax won't melt. Over-stirring cools your beeswax and will keep it from melting.

Your salve is ready to pour when the wax has melted completely into the oil. Wipe off the underside of your oil bowl, especially the rim, and then carefully pour your salve into small jars.

Put lids and labels on the jars only after the salve has set and cooled completely.

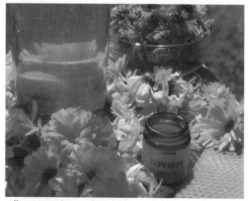

All you need to make a salve—oil, dried or fresh calendula, and beeswax—and one finished jar.

A FEW OTHER HERBAL SALVES

Any of the herbs suggested under "Which herb should I use?" (page 16) will work well for single-herb salves. Salves made with strongly scented peppermint or using canola oil require extra beeswax to set properly.

Here are a few pleasant blends to try, and one spicy salve:

- *The gardener's salve*, good for painful muscles and dirt-roughened skin, combines oils from meadowsweet (or balsam poplar buds) and calendula flowers (or *Plantago* plantain leaves).

- *Ouch I fell* (or perhaps *Head over heels*) is tailor-made for for kids and athletes—meadowsweet (or balsam poplar buds) for pain, calendula (or plantain leaf) for small wounds and abrasions, and St. John's wort, extremely good for bruises and swellings from trauma.

- *Warming* salve is useful where winters (and feet) are cold. It also helps with muscle aches and can be rubbed on the chest and back against coughs. Use these ingredients:

  2 cups (500 ml) oil
  1.5 ounces (40 g) powdered cayenne
  0.5 ounces (15 g) powdered mustard
  0.5 ounces (15 g) powdered ginger
  4 ounces (10 g) powdered black pepper
  beeswax as needed

Make sure your ground spices are fresh. The salve starts to warm nicely about 15 minutes after application.
Be sure to wash your hands with soap after using this salve to avoid getting any in your eyes (or other delicate spots).

• *Keep-away* tar salve will repel stinging insects that navigate by smell: stir 1 teaspoon pine tar into a quart (liter) of oil or herbal oil, and make your salve from the blend. This has a pleasant scent and works much as resin salves do. You can try it on almost anything.

PROBLEMS WITH OIL-BASED SALVES

• Your salve is too soft, or even runny. You didn't use enough beeswax. You could re-melt your salve and add more beeswax, but that's messy and a lot of work. I suggest you measure things more precisely in the future.

• Your salve can be too hard. You used too much beeswax. Again, you can re-melt your salve and add more oil, but that, too, is messy and a lot of work. Measure accurately.

• Your salve supports mold. This can happen if water got into the salve at some point, or if your dried herb wasn't dry enough.

• You find insect legs or wings at the bottom of a salve jar. If you didn't strain your melted raw beeswax through cheesecloth, you may end up with a bee's knee or wing in your wax.

• The insides of your salve jars are "messy." You didn't let the salve set solidly before you added lids and labels. The runny contents splashed all over, and then set that way.

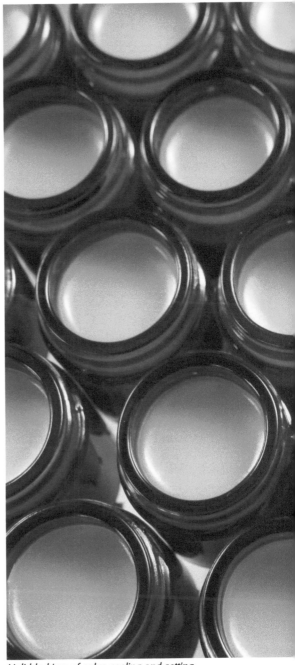

Unlidded jars of salve cooling and setting.

23

TINCTURES

Fresh herbs are best stored as tinctures or alcohol extracts.

A (surprisingly small) dose of just 15 to 30 drops taken one to three times a day is normal for tinctures made from both fresh and dried herb material. Some fresh-herb tinctures require even smaller doses—just one to three drops as needed can be enough. If this is the case, you may notice the tincture's effects within 30 to 60 seconds of ingesting it, because it's been absorbed by the mouth's membranes, bypassing the digestive system. Thus absorbed into the oral mucosa, it passes directly into the bloodstream.

TINCTURE STABILITY

Most herbal tinctures will remain effective for years, especially if you store them at room temperature in dark glass bottles.

A few more fragile herbs, however, won't last long even as tincture. For instance, shepherd's purse must be tinctured afresh each and every year, especially if you're after the herb's oxytocin-enhancing effect.

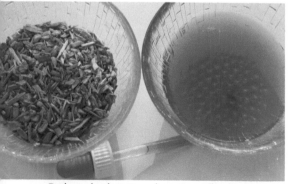

Barberry bush roots make a nice yellow tincture.

A SIMPLE TINCTURE

This is also called simpler's tincture.

From fresh herb

Green parts: cut your herb material into 1-inch (2–3 cm) lengths.

Roots: wash and cut in 1/4-inch (5 mm) slices, with 1-inch (2–3 cm) lengths, as needed.

Put as much fresh herb as possible into a clean glass jar and cover with your menstruum—that is, the alcohol you tincture with.

For fresh herb, use a strong alcohol: 95 percent is best (grain or ethyl alcohol, "ethanol"), 80 percent is fine, 60 percent will work, 40 percent is so-so.

"Proof" is the percentage doubled. Thus, 95 percent is 190 proof, 40 percent is 80 proof, and so on.

Screw the lid on tightly and leave the jar in a dark cool corner for a few weeks.

Strain, bottle, and label. The label should state the name of the herb, how you made the tincture, the strength of alcohol, and the date of the tincture. For instance, "Simpler's tincture of fresh St. John's wort, Stroh Rum 80 %, July 2021."

Store your bottles in a dark cool spot.

From dried herb

The basic recipe is the same as for the fresh herb, but for dried herb 60 percent alcohol is best.

40 percent will work, but generally will require larger doses to be effective.

A MORE OFFICIAL TINCTURE

You'll need both measuring cups and a kitchen scale if you want to make a tincture that stays uniformly consistent in quality from batch to batch and year to year, and as strong as commercial tincture.

From fresh herb

Take 1 part (by weight) fresh herb to 2 parts (by volume) of strong alcohol (95 percent)—that is, 1:2 95 %. For example:

 4 ounces (100 g) fresh herb
 8 fluid ounces (200 ml) 95 % (190 proof) grain alcohol

Put herb material in a jar and cover completely with alcohol. Lid tightly, and leave your tincture-to-be in a dark spot for two to four weeks.

Strain, bottle, and label: include the herb's name, where you picked it, the tincture strength, and the date. (Example: "Fresh carrot seed and flowers, Grandma's yard, 1:2 95 % Everclear, August 2021.")

From dried herb

Take 1 part (by weight) dried herb to 5 parts (by volume) of grain alcohol (60 percent)—1:5 60 %. For example:

 4 ounces (100 g) dried herb
 20 fluid ounces (500 ml) 120 proof grain alcohol (60 %)

Add both to a jar. Make sure the alcohol covers the herb. Close the lid tightly, and leave your tincture-to-be in a dark spot for two to four weeks.

Strain, bottle, and label with herb name, where you picked it, alcohol strength, and date (example: "Dried California poppy, my garden, 1:2 60 % Everclear, September 2021").

ALCOHOL STRENGTH AND TINCTURE QUALITY

To make a tincture, some water must be present, either in the herb or in the menstruum itself.

Because fresh herb is 80 to 90 percent water, if you use 95 percent alcohol, you'll get a tincture that's as strong as it can get. But because 190 proof alcohol is illegal in some places, you may have to be satisfied with 80 percent alcohol for your tinctures. If 60 percent is what you can get, use that.

Dried herb material contains only 10 to 15 percent water, so if you used 95 percent alcohol to tincture it, you'd extract only its alcohol-soluble constituents. But the water-soluble ones are just as important! Instead, use a menstruum of 60 percent alcohol (that is, 40 percent water) for dried herb.

A weaker alcohol—for instance, 60 percent for fresh herb or 40 percent for dried—yields a weaker tincture, and thus the need for larger doses.

If you have only vodka or the like (32 to 40 percent alcohol), make your tincture from dried herb. If you don't, the alcohol content of your finished fresh-herb tincture will be lower than 12 percent, and that means your tincture can spoil (and your bottles or jars may explode in your cupboard!).

Filling a jar

Make sure your menstruum covers the herb. If some of the herb stays above the liquid, weight it down with a few smooth clean stones or a small glass (or undecorated plastic) jar or cup. Once the herb is covered, screw the lid on tightly.

25

HERBAL VINEGARS

The taste and color of herbal vinegars fade over time or with exposure to light. That astonishing pink of your chives flower vinegar will turn a dull yellow after a year, even though you've kept the bottle in a dark cupboard. If you keep such a beautiful vinegar on the table, the color will fade even faster.

So use up your vinegars! You'll be glad of their taste and colors.

The best herbal vinegars for cooking include chives, horseradish, the mints, rosemary, sage, thyme, and garlic.

Try making your herbal vinegar from a mineral-rich herb, such as stinging nettles, lady's mantle, the green parts of oats, red raspberry leaf, or field horsetail. Add 1 to 3 teaspoons of your finished vinegar to a glass of water, and you've met your mineral requirements for the day.

If you don't like the taste of your herbal vinegar, you'll be relieved to know that vinegars are great for cleaning the tiles in your bathroom. Years ago I ended up

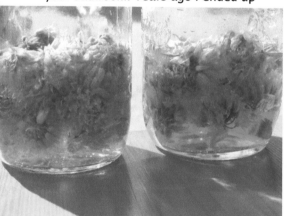

Flowers of chives in diluted white vinegar and apple cider vinegar.

using my lavender vinegar for just that, as the taste was all too floral for my cooking.

Diluted white vinegar (to 5 percent acetic acid) works as well as apple cider or wine vinegars in the following formulas.

HOW TO MAKE AN HERBAL VINEGAR

12 fluid ounces (350 ml) apple cider vinegar
fresh herbs

Fill a jar with herbs, cover with vinegar, and leave for two to four weeks in a dark cupboard.

Strain into a pretty glass bottle, add one twig of each herb you used (for decoration), and label (example: "Basil and thyme vinegar, July 2021"). Use as a condiment.

To use instead of an herbal tea or tincture: 1–3 teaspoons to a glass of water. Drink one to two glasses a day.

CHIVES FLOWER VINEGAR

chives flowers
apple cider vinegar

Fill a jar with chives flowers, cover with vinegar, and leave in a dark spot for two to four weeks. Strain, bottle, and label.

The flavor of this vinegar will be oniony and sweetish, the color a light "old rose." Using a diluted white vinegar instead of apple cider vinegar here yields a stunning shocking pink.

If you add chives flowers back to your finished vinegar for decoration, make sure no ants are hiding in them! Ants love chives.

HERBAL SYRUPS

Sugary herbal products such as syrups are good for dry coughs because sugar increases mucus secretion. Don't use syrups for digestive troubles, however, because sugar interferes with digestion.

Like all simple carbs and sweets, of course, syrups should be taken in moderation.

Because an herbal syrup will stay liquid in the freezer, you can keep it there for years on end. But out of sight out of mind—you may remember it only when you clean the freezer out, and not when someone near and dear starts to cough.

(In 2000 I noticed that the juniper berry syrup I'd made in 1989 had changed into a frozen jelly. After I moved it to the fridge, this jelly separated into two layers, and the upper layer grew mold within a week. Just think, if I had moved only a part of the syrup to the fridge back in 2000, I could now report what a frozen syrup looks like after more than 20 years in the freezer!)

If you keep your syrup refrigerated, it will grow crystals as months go by—especially if you open the jar from time to time—but at least you'll remember to use it when someone needs it (or when you make pancakes).

HOW TO MAKE AN HERBAL SYRUP

The beginning:

1 quart (liter) water
fresh herb material enough that the water covers it
or 0.5–0.7 ounces (15–20 g) dried aboveground parts
or 1 cup (250 ml) fresh or dried roots or bark, in smallish pieces

Put the herb in a saucepan and cover it with the water. Bring to a boil and simmer for 15 to 25 minutes. Strain.

If you want a stronger syrup, you can now add more herb to the same liquid. Again, bring to a boil, simmer for 15 to 25 minutes, and strain.

Next, you can either evaporate your liquid slowly over low heat until only three-quarters of a cup (200 ml) remains, or, bored with the interminable waiting, pour off that amount right away.

But don't discard the rest of the liquid: if this particular batch turns out to be perfect, you'll want to make another immediately.

The finish:

3/4 cup (200 ml) of above liquid
13 ounces (425 g, or about a pound) granulated sugar

Add sugar to the liquid, set the heat to as close to none at all as you can, and stir your mix until the sugar has dissolved. Pour the syrup into glass jars, close with a tight-fitting lid, and label (example: "Herbal syrup, blue spruce and mugo pine spring growth, June 2021. 1 tsp. as needed for coughs").

DARK SPRUCE SYRUP

4-1/2 quarts (5 l, or a little more than a gallon) of the spring growth of spruce
water
sugar

Rinse the spruce shoots, put them in a large cooking pot, and cover them with water. Leave overnight.

Boil for an hour or two. Leave overnight.

Strain and measure the liquid. Add a pound (500 g) of sugar to each quart (liter) of liquid. Simmer until the liquid is a clear, dark red.

Let a few drops of your sugary liquid drip onto a cold surface and pull the broad bottom of a spoon through it. If the liquid reunites, it's not quite done yet.

Pour into jars and label (example: "Dark spruce shoot syrup, June 2021. 1 tsp. as needed for cough").

GOOD HERBS FOR HERBAL SYRUPS

These herbs and herb combinations make nice syrups:

- 1 part thyme, 2 parts hyssop, 4 parts peppermint. Excellent for coughs, but so tasty that it's all gone by the time anybody needs it.
- Peppermint is nice by itself, too. Add some to refreshing summery drinks.
- Dandelion flowers. This makes a tasty syrup, but it has no medicinal uses. Don't bother removing the green flower parts.
- Shoots of spruce, pine, or fir, or berries of a nontoxic juniper. Good for coughs and to season desserts. Syrup made from a mix of blue spruce and mountain pine shoots has a tangy, "forest-y" flavor.
- Elecampane roots. Excellent for coughs, especially if digestive problems are also present.
- Angelica flowers, roots, or fresh seed. Angelicas need something sour: add a dash of lemon juice, rhubarb, or citric acid to your syrup.
- Plantain (Plantago species) leaf. Great for coughs.
- Sweet flag (Acorus calamus) root. Also good for coughs.
- Hollyhock flowers. These make for intriguing colours but have absolutely no flavor. Make some, and let your dinner guests try to guess what this sticky liquid might be!

PROBLEMS WITH SYRUPS

Herbal syrups are notoriously difficult to make—perhaps the herb is more or less watery than last year, or the water is less or more watery—uh, no, not that. But getting a perfect syrup is tricky.

If your finished syrup crystallizes readily, it's too sugary. You let too much water evaporate. Use less sugar in the next batch.

If your syrup spoils or grows moldy, it's too watery. You let too little water evaporate. Use more sugar in the next batch.

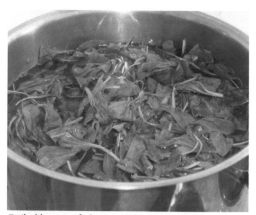

Boiled leaves of plantain (Plantago). The syrup is made from just the liquid.

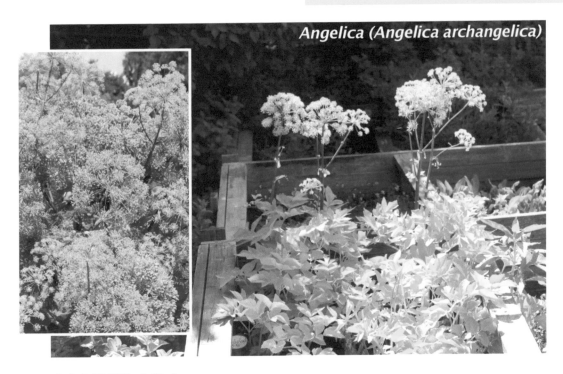

Angelica (Angelica archangelica)

ANGELICA

The one herb that's been introduced to Central Europe from far-northern countries.

Angelica archangelica: Also called archangel, garden angelica, wild celery

Family: Carrot family (umbellifers), *Apiaceae (Umbelliferae)*

Biennial: Harvest spring to fall (root), fall (seed). (If you can't get this species, you can use other Angelica species.)

Habitat: Angelica grows near water.

Cultivation: Angelica seeds are at their best in autumn; sown then, most will germinate. If you wait until spring, few if any will.

As a biennial, angelica will flower in its second summer and die after it sets seed. If you cut the flower stalks as they appear, though, you can turn angelica into a short-lived perennial.

The flower stalk can grow to 5 feet (1.5 m) or more. The leaf mass will stay at a bit under 3 feet (1 m).

Appearance: Angelica flowers are yellowish green. The flower head is made up of globes-within-a-globe; that is, the single flowers form many small globes, which in turn form a head-sized globe. One flower stalk can sport several such heads, and one plant can have several flower stalks. The leaves are larger and less finely divided than those of our other wild species, wild angelica.

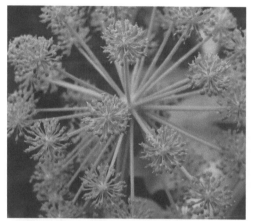

Angelica (Angelica archangelica) in full flower.

Look-alikes: Be careful. A lot of umbellifers resemble angelica:

- Giant hogweed (*Heracleum mantegazzianum*) is much larger than angelica; its flowerhead is flat and the flowers are white. Giant hogweed sap can cause severe burns.

- Cow parsnip or hogweed (*Heracleum sphondylium*) is a little smaller than angelica. The leaves and stems are coarse, the flowerheads flat, and the flowers white.

- The young leaves of goutweed (*Aegopodium podagraria*) can look like angelica. Goutweed doesn't have a taproot, but rooting runners. Don't pull up all your young angelicas thinking they're goutweed!

- Wild angelica (*Angelica sylvestris*) is far more delicate than garden angelica. Its flowers are off-white, the smaller flower clusters are halfglobes, and the flowerhead looks like a flattened half-globe.

- Water hemlock (*Cicuta virosa*) grows in wet soils. It's a lot smaller than angelica; the general color is bluish green, the flowerheads are flat and the flowers white. Water hemlock is deadly.

- Poison hemlock (*Conium maculatum*) looks more like a fern than like angelica, but I include it here because poison hemlock is deadly.

If you can't tell angelica from water hemlock, grow it. That way you can be sure.

Important constituents: Essential oils, angelic acid, bitters, coumarins (not blood-thinning dicoumaroles), oils, tannins

PICKING AND PROCESSING

Dig the roots before the plant flowers.

Because the roots of biennial plants must anchor their flower stalks, they grow woody once the plant flowers. Also, the active constituents in the first-year roots get used up when the plant flowers.

Biennials (and their roots) die once the plants set seed.

Rinse the roots outdoors, pull off various contorted parts (but use them, too!), and then scrub them with a brush. You needn't remove the root bark, but do get rid of small stones, soil, and earthworms.

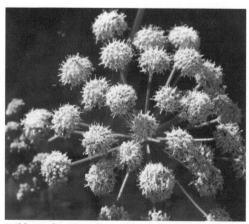

Wild angelica (Angelica sylvestris) in full flower.

Cut the washed roots into quarter-inch (5 mm) slices, and dry them in a dehydrator set below 95 °F (35 °C) or on a cotton cloth or bedsheet. They're done when they don't bend, but break. Label (example: "Angelica roots, my garden, September 2021"), and store the dried slices in an airtight jar in a dark cupboard.

Dried angelica root keeps for about two years. If the taste has become mild—almost tasty—the root has lost its effect; throw it on your compost heap.

Harvest the seeds from the largest seed heads when the stems are still a little green. If you wait too long the seeds will fall off. Spread them to dry on an absorbant surface such as paper towels.

EFFECTS AND USES

Angelica is excellent for menstrual pain. It works even for the pain of endometriosis. Chew a piece of root and relax. The pain is already gone.

Chewing the root works for normal menstrual discomfort, too, but for that you can use a tea or tincture of angelica, as well.

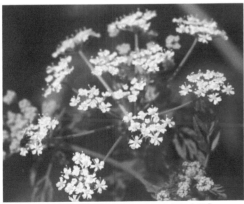

Poison hemlock (Conium maculatum) in full flower.

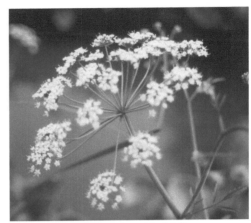

Water hemlock (Cicuta virosa) in full flower.

Both roots and seeds help with digestive problems such as loss of appetite, gut cramps, and flatulence. Either works as tea, tincture, or chewed out of hand.

For chronic digestive upset, take angelica about 20 minutes before every meal.

If you feel nauseated but can't seem to vomit, chew on a few seeds, and drink water. Consider making an electrolyte beverage:

  1 cup (250 ml) warm water
  1 teaspoon salt
  1 tablespoon sugar

Mix; drink.

Angelica also is effective for respiratory problems, especially coughs.

A hot tea of angelica seeds helps you sweat. Drink the tea if you feel like you're getting the flu, if you have a cough, or if you have a low fever.

Externally, a compress of the roots helps relieve arthritic joint pain and the like.

BITTERS

Bitter foods and herbs strengthen the digestion. A bitter taste on the tongue stimulates more saliva, which leads to more secretions of the esophagus, which leads to more secretions in the stomach lining, which leads to more secretions in the pancreas and secretions of bile in the liver, which leads to more secretions in the intestines.

The digestion as a whole works more smoothly and the appetite is stimulated.

Bitter herbs are divided into

- simple bitters: dandelion, chicory, burdock, gentian;
- aromatic bitters: angelica, calamus or sweet flag, mugwort, coffee, juniper, yarrow;
- sour bitters: grapefruit, ginger.

Aromatic bitters such as angelica help with both a weakened digestion and the gut-pinching pain that comes with that weakening.

Sour bitters don't necessarily taste bitter.

The most effective bitter is both aromatic and sour—an angelica or mugwort vinegar, for example.

Angelica root decoction

1 teaspoon dried roots
1 cup (250 ml) cold water

Put the herb in a saucepan and add water. Bring to a boil, simmer for 10 minutes, cool, and strain.

Drink 2 fluid ounces (50 ml) of this tea up to four times a day.

Angelica chewed

Chew a few seeds or a piece of root, as needed.

Angelica root necklace

Use one or more of the more decorative dried root bits as a necklace.

You can then either just admire the result or chew on a piece of root as needed.

Angelica tea

1 teaspoon dried seeds or roots
1 cup (250 ml) boiling water

Pour boiling water over the herb and steep until the liquid has cooled. Strain and drink two or three cups a day.

Angelica root maceration

1/2 teaspoon dried roots
1 cup (250 ml) cold water

Pour water into a jar, add the root, steep for eight hours, and strain. Sip throughout the day.

Angelica root tincture

From fresh root:

4 ounces (100 g) fresh angelica root in thin slices, sticks, or bits
8 fluid ounces (200 ml) 190 proof grain alcohol (95 %)

From dried root:

4 ounces (100 g) dried roots in thin slices, sticks, or bits
20 fluid ounces (500 ml) 130 proof grain alcohol (65 %)

Put the roots in a glass jar, cover with the alcohol, and close the lid tightly. Steep for two to four weeks. Strain, bottle, and label (example, fresh: "Angelica root, 1:2 95 %, 9.2021, Granddad's forest"; example, dried: "Angelica root, 1:5 65 %, 04.2021, my garden").

Dosage is 30–60 drops, up to four times a day.

Angelica seed tincture

From fresh seed:

  4 ounces (100 g) fresh seed
  8 fluid ounces (200 ml) 190 proof grain
   alcohol (95 %)

From dried seed:

  4 ounces (100 g) dried seed
  20 fluid ounces (500 ml) 130 proof grain
   alcohol (65 %)

Put the seed in a glass jar, cover with the alcohol, and close the lid tightly. Steep for two to four weeks. Strain, bottle, and label (example, fresh: "Angelica seed, 1:2 95 %, 09.2021, my own yard"; example, dried: "Angelica seed, 1:5 65 %, 04.2021, Granddad's garden").

Dosage is 10–30 drops, up to four times a day.

FOOD USES

If you wish to bring angelica to your table, remember two things:

1. Angelica has a strong taste; use small amounts.

2. Angelica is bitter and needs something sour to balance it.

So do add green seeds, young leaves, young stems, and young flowers to your rhubarb pie, make a tea and serve it with some lemon juice, or freeze young angelica and use it later on to spice up your sour apple sauce.

But if you forget to include some sourness, angelica tastes terrible.

WARNINGS

Because angelica enhances pelvic circulation, especially when it's fresh, you should avoid it if you are pregnant. Also, those with sensitive skin may get a rash from the juice of angelica. This is usually short-lived and nothing to worry about.

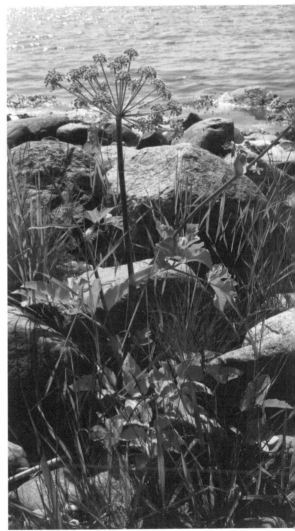

An angelica growing wild on the shore of the Baltic sea.

PAINFUL MENSES

The roots of angelica (*Angelica archangelica*) and its cousin wild angelica (*Angelica sylvestris*) are without a doubt among our best herbs for treating menstrual cramps.

These roots taste so bad you're unlikely to take them unless your menstrual pain is severe. In that case, don't potter around the kitchen making a tea. Instead, keep a small container of angelica root bits in your purse to chew on. If the root isn't too old, the pain will stop.

Don't go digging angelicas if you don't know your umbellifers. There are deadly look-alikes in this family.

Dig the roots after the plant's first summer, but before it starts to grow the flower stalk its second summer. Wash the roots, slice them, and spread the slices to dry on a cotton cloth or old bedsheet. After a week to 10 days, the roots are dry (they break rather than bend) and can be stored in an airtight jar. Label (example: "Angelica root, September 2021").

The root keeps for about two years, but older roots often can provide relief for milder menstrual cramps.

The root of calamus or sweet flag (*Acorus calamus*) can be used instead of angelica root. Dried calamus root keeps for years if it's stored airtight in a dark cupboard.

For long-term help with menstrual pain, take magnesium and vitamin B (especially B6).

More than half the ladies suffering from painful menses find relief after taking supplemental magnesium or including magnesium-rich foods in their diet.

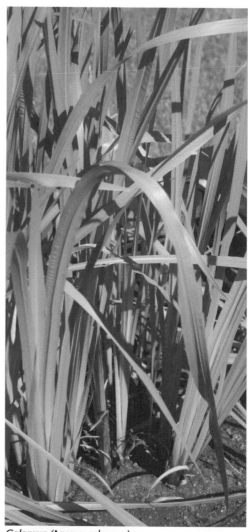

Calamus (Acorus calamus).

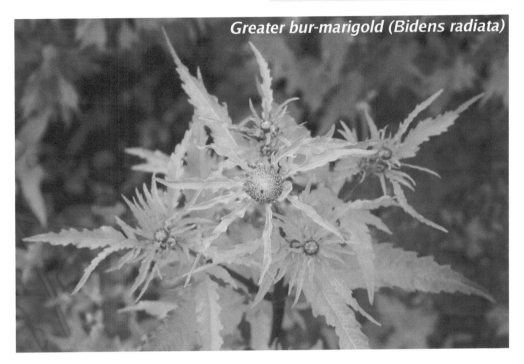

Greater bur-marigold (Bidens radiata)

BEGGARTICKS

A weed that's very good at hiding—but you'll find the seeds easily enough in your dog's fur.

Bidens species: Including

- Nodding bur-marigold (*Bidens cernua*); also called beggar-ticks, stick-tight
- Greater bur-marigold (*Bidens radiata*)
- Three-lobed beggarticks (*Bidens tripartita*); also called water agrimony, bastard agrimony, swamp beggar-ticks

Family: Daisy family, *Asteraceae*

Annual: Harvest in late summer.

Habitat: Beggarticks are easiest to spot on newly cleared soil, where competing species haven't really taken off yet. Here, one beggarticks plant can be 18 inches (about a half-meter) tall and 36 inches (1 m) in diameter.

Cutting a single plant can get you a year's supply.

In lush meadows, on the other hand, the plant can be next to invisible: in one such field I collected every plant I could find every day for two weeks, and ended up with a single armful of beggarticks.

Dog-owners know beggarticks from the dark brown, flat, barbed seeds their pet brings home in its fur.

Bidens species can be found growing throughout the U.S. and Canada and most of Europe and southern Scandinavia.

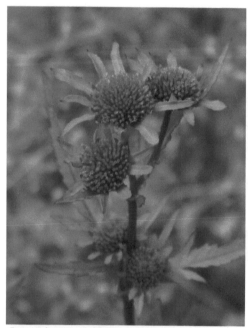

*Greater bur-marigold (*Bidens radiata*) in seed.*

Cultivation: You can use any species of *Bidens*, including those grown as summer flowers, provided they're grown organically.

Appearance: It's easy to identify beggarticks from its seeds, which grab hold of your woollen sweater, and from the leaves surrounding its flowers in that unique beggarticks pattern.

Our Finnish wild species lack petals; the flowers are either brownish green or greenish yellow.

Important constituents: Tannins, flavonoids, essential oil

PICKING AND PROCESSING

Cut beggarticks a bit above the base, or pull up the plant roots and all.

Pick plants in full flower and dry them in hanging bundles or in a dehydrator. Remove the thickest stems from the dried herbs.

EFFECTS AND USES

Beggarticks moistens pelvic mucosa, as well as mucous membranes of the digestive and respiratory tracts. I use it in all urinary tract infections and in benign enlargement of the prostate (benign prostatic hyperplasia, BPHP).

The herb also helps with the itching anus that sometimes accompanies BPHP.

Take a tea of beggarticks if you have dry mucous membranes.

Beggarticks works for urinary tract infections, soothing mucosa, relieving pain, and halting light bleeding. For more severe bleeding, see a doctor as soon as possible. (Another herb for bleeding is shepherd's purse, *Capsella bursa-pastoris*—page 132. Mallows—page 50—also moisten mucous membranes.)

Beggarticks help with recurrent urinary tract infections, too, but try to nail down the reason for the problem. Check your sugar intake, try to lower your stress levels and drink enough water.

Use beggarticks for gout; it assists the kidneys in removing uric acid from the blood.

The plant is great for hay fever, as it soothes the mucous membranes. If you also take stinging nettles during the summer, you may just get by without your hay-fever medication.

I give beggarticks (or mallows) for digestive upset, too, but I also try to determine the source of the problem. Which food might be a culprit?

Its effect on mucous membranes becomes obvious in the way it works for a dripping nose, continual light cough, and neverending throat irritation. I also use it in leucorrhea (a white vaginal discharge), but for that I recommend B vitamins, as well.

A tea of beggarticks is tasty. You can drink it daily for months on end, if you wish, so pick enough of it!

Tea of beggarticks

  1–2 teaspoons dried beggarticks
  1 cup (250 ml) boiling water

Pour boiling water over the herb, steep for 10 minutes, and strain. Drink three to four cups a day.

WARNINGS

If you get a skin rash when you touch chamomile or mugwort, you can, in theory, also get a skin rash from beggarticks.

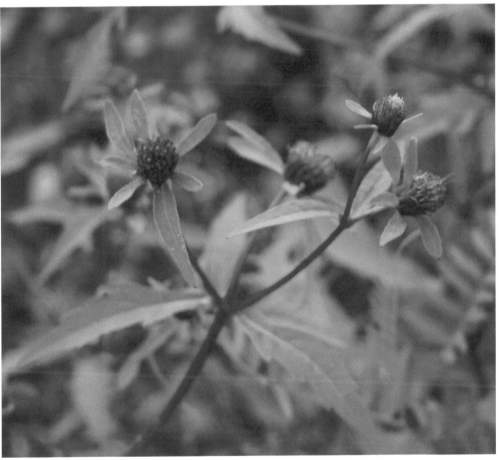

Threelobed beggarticks (Bidens tripartita).

CARROT-FAMILY CARMINATIVE PLANTS

Did you eat too much over the holidays?

Do you have that queasy feeling that comes after eating fast food, with its rancid fats?

Have you eaten a tad too many raw onions, and now your digestive tract protests with twinges and flatulence?

Simply chew a few seeds of an edible carrot-family plant.

You'll find relief within minutes of chomping just five or ten caraway seeds. Other species that work include aniseed, fennel, coriander, cumin, dill, celeriac, lovage, angelica, and even carrot seeds.

The green seeds of sweet cicely can be effective, too; its ripe seeds lack scent and flavor, and so can't soothe digestion.

Avoid the seeds of giant hogweed. They smell terrible, and the sap is extremely sun-sensitizing; you can burn badly where it gets on your skin.

Avoid the seeds of toxic look-alikes. If you don't know your angelicas from your cicutas, leave both of them in place.

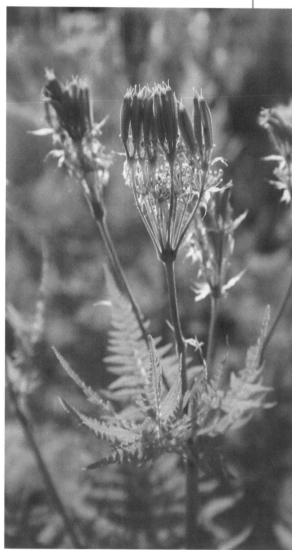

*The green seeds of sweet cicely (*Myrrhis odorata*) taste of anise candy.*

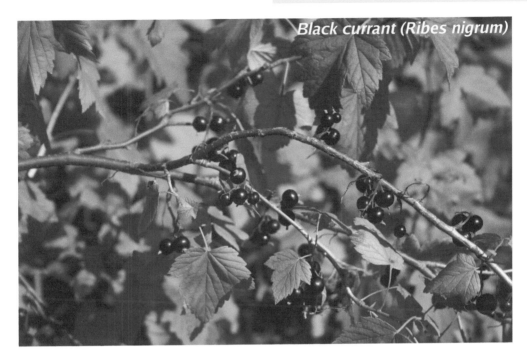

Black currant (Ribes nigrum)

BLACK CURRANT

A delicious berry, tasty leaves, and buds that help treat allergies.

Ribes nigrum: Also called European black currant

Family: Gooseberry family, *Grossulariaceae*

Perennial: Harvest flower buds and leaf buds in spring, berries in summer, and leaves from late spring to early fall.

Habitat: Here in Finland black currant grows wild along lake shores and riverbanks, and among deciduous trees. Wild bushes are less lush than their cousins and yield fewer berries. Plants growing with wet feet are also more vulnerable to powdery mildew early in summer.

Cultivation: Select a mildew-proof cultivar.

Although planting in a sunny spot makes for sweeter berries, you risk damage in the early spring when the sun's heat may open the buds while the ground is still frozen.

You'll get a smallish bush if you grow it in clay soil.

Remove dead and damaged branches in spring.

Many U.S. states used to restrict the cultivation of black currant. Some northern states still do. Check with your local ag agent or nursery if you're not sure.

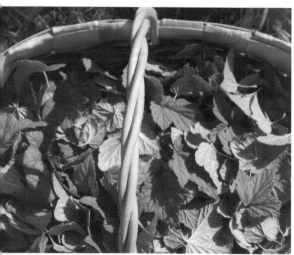

The leaf of black currant (Ribes nigrum).

Look-alikes: Other currants. Don't use unscented leaf for allergies (or as a tasty tidbit). It's possible to mistake the berry of golden currant for black currant, but black currant doesn't have golden currant's 1–2-inch (3 cm) flower. The berry of golden currant is less tasty than that of black currant.

Important constituents: Flavonoids, vitamins A, C, and some Bs, plant acids, sugars, pectin, tannins, potassium (berry); essential oils, tannins, vitamin C (leaves)

PICKING AND PROCESSING

Herbal medicine mostly makes use of the hot juice. The less sugar in the juice, the better (but the juice needn't be undrinkably sour).

The leaves are tasty in sandwich spreads, as seasoning, in herbal teas, and made into a lemony syrup similar to that prepared from black elder flowers (hard to come by up my way).

Gather leaves and leafy tops from summer to fall, as long as they don't have fungal diseases or too much insect damage.

Alternate leaf-gathering years with berry-picking ones, according to the rhythm of the plant. Pick leaves when flowers and berries are less abundant and when leaf growth is lusher.

Spread the leaves and tops you picked indoors out of the light and store in glass jars as soon as they're completely dry.

Pick flower and leaf buds and young leaves in spring. Use them as you use full-grown leaves, or tincture them.

EFFECTS AND USES

Hot black currant juice is good for the earliest symptoms of respiratory tract infection. The hot juice is effective once the flu hits, too. It's ideal for the feverish; those with stuffy noses need their vitamins, flavonoids, and hot drinks.

The berries are diuretic and taken hot can bring on sweating.

Because the berries are so high in flavonoids, they help strengthen capillaries.

Historically, black currant was used for joint troubles, and the berries were called "gout berries"; eat 4 ounces (100 grams) daily, or drink a half-cup of diluted juice every day. (Black cherries, strawberries, and black elderberries have also been called "gout berries.")

Black currant juice, berries, jam, and the like all help with sore throat and hoarseness—gargled or eaten, as the case may be. If you have frozen berries, you can make a hot "tea" from them.

The very young leaves and flower and leaf buds can be tinctured for treating allergies, eczemas, and asthma.

The *Flora Fennica* of 1866 mentions the use of the twigs and young leaves as a tea for joint aches and long-term coughs.

Decoction of black currant berries

1 tablespoon berries
1 cup (250 ml) cold water

Put berries and water in a saucepan, bring to a boil, simmer for 10 minutes, and strain. Drink as much as you like.

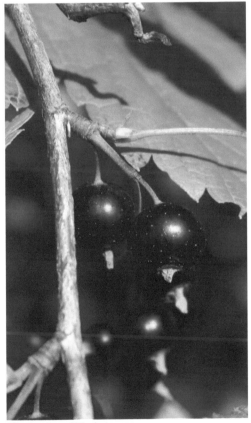

The berries of black currant.

Black currant leaf tea

1–2 teaspoons dried or fresh leaves
1 cup (250 ml) boiling water

Pour boiling water over the herb, steep for 5 minutes, and strain. Drink up to three cups a day for joint aches, diarrhea, and allergies.

If you steep the leaves too long, the tannins render the tea almost undrinkable. Brew another cup.

Black currant bud tincture

From fresh buds:

1/3 ounce (10 g) fresh flower buds or leaf buds
8 fluid ounces (200 ml) 190 proof grain alcohol (95 %)

From dried buds:

1/3 ounce (10 g) dried flower buds or leaf buds
8 fluid ounces (200 ml) 100 proof grain alcohol (50 %)

Put the buds into a glass jar, cover with alcohol, and close the lid tightly. Steep two to four weeks, strain, bottle, and label (example, fresh: "Black currant, fresh buds, 1:20 95 %, June 2021, Granddad's garden"; example, dried: "Black currant, dried buds, 1:20 50 %, August 2021, front yard").

Dosage is two to five drops under your tongue as needed, or one or two times a day. This is so-called "gemmotherapy" —a very weak tincture of plant buds in full growth.

FOOD USES

The berries yield juice, jam, jelly and other delicacies. Black currant juice can be used in place of red wine for nonalcoholic mulled wine.

The leaves can be used in pickling cucumbers. Use the young leaves on your sandwiches, too!

Black currant leaves make a tasty, lemony syrup. And you can use them to spice up your home-brewed beers, wines, and meads.

Because you can make a flavorful tea from the leaves, buds, and bark, don't throw pruned branches onto the compost heap until you've removed everything usable from them.

Add the leaves to fruit salads and herbal sandwich spreads.

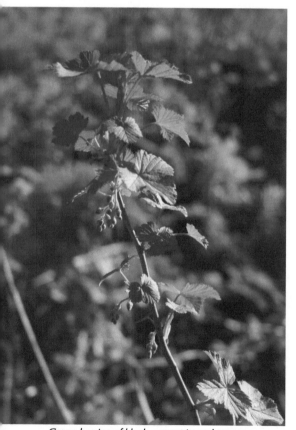

Green berries of black currant in early summer.

Nonalcoholic mulled wine

1 cup (250 ml) black currant berry juice
1 quart (liter) water
1–2 cinnamon sticks, 2 or 3 inches (5–8 cm) long
half a split vanilla pod
4–6 cloves
seeds of 4–5 cardamom pods

Bring the water to a boil, add the juice and spices, and steep on very low heat for 15 minutes. Serve with crushed or sliced almonds and raisins.

Black currant sugar

half an ounce (15 g) dried black currant leaves
1 cup (250 ml) sugar

Combine in a blender and whirl the mixture until the leaf is powdered. Store in an airtight glass jar. Yum!

Black currant leaf syrup

5 quarts (5 liters) black currant leaves
8 quarts (8 liters) water
2 ounces (50 g) citric acid
2 pounds (1 kg) sugar

Layer the leaves in a saucepan with the citric acid. Add boiling water. Steep overnight.

The following morning, strain out the leaves and stir to dissolve the sugar in the liquid.

The syrup will keep for a few days in the refrigerator; you can also freeze it.

Serve diluted with water, 1:3 or 1:5.

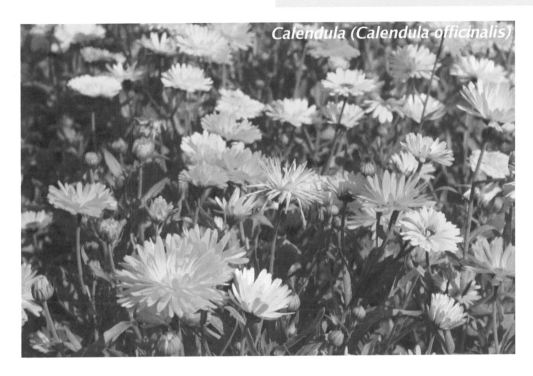

Calendula (Calendula officinalis)

CALENDULA

This brightly colored garden beauty is an excellent wound healer.

Calendula officinalis: Also called pot marigold

Family: Daisy (*Asteraceae; Compositae: Tubuliflorae*)

Annual: Harvest in its flowering period—early summer to frost.

Habitat: The original calendula species, from Egypt and the Mediterranean, is pale yellow and small-flowered. It has been cultivated all over Europe since the 12th century and traveled with European settlers to North America.

Cultivation: Use seeds from the previous year's calendula, or buy fresh seeds.

Plants from seeds you gather yourself get less and less showy as years go by.

Sow in a sunny spot after danger of frost has passed. Harvest from summer to fall.

Appearance: Calendula can grow to about 18 inches (50 cm) and flowers from the end of June until first frost. Flower color ranges from pale yellow to dark orange.

Important constituents: Essential oils, glycosides, flavonoids, bitters, organic acids

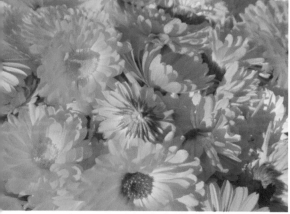

Bright orange calendula flowers.

PICKING AND PROCESSING

Once it's completely open, remove the whole flower, even if you want just the petals. This will keep your calendula plant blooming.

Spread a cotton cloth, such as a bed sheet, on a layer of newspapers out of the light, and arrange your calendula blossoms on it. If you picked them on a rainy day, tap the flowers dry between sheets before spreading them to dry—or use a salad spinner. A too-damp, too-large flower will go moldy before it's dry.

You may notice a green caterpillar living in all too many flowers. Because it's the same green as the flower, it's next to impossible to see. They continue producing dung on the drying flowers, though, and so you can locate them via their byproducts: if you notice droppings, you know the caterpillar that produced them must be in that flower. The larger the droppings, the larger the caterpillar.

You can always dry your calendula in a dehydrator, but in that case the caterpillars will end up dying on the racks.

Dry calendula at lowish temperatures—95 °F (35 °C) at the most; any higher and the dried herb develops a very strong smell.

Properly dried calendula is strongly colored and has a mild calendula scent.

Old, useless calendula is very pale and smelly.

EFFECTS AND USES

Used externally, calendula speeds healing of wounds on the skin and mucous membranes and reduces the formation of scar tissue.

Use it to treat all kinds of abrasions, eczema, small wounds, and minor burns. It also helps with psoriasis (but in that case check your diet, too: do you get enough vitamins D and B?).

Because calendula slightly enhances local blood circulation, it's nice for bruises and sprains. And it's absolutely astonishing for long-standing tiny wounds: a hint of a dab of the oil or salve, and the wound is no more.

Dr. Gerhard Madaus, in his *Lehrbuch der Biologischen Heilmittel* (1938), describes calendula's effect on a years-old itchy wound at the stump end of an amputation: as long as the stump was washed with calendula soap, leaving the suds on to dry, and calendula salve was massaged into the area, the wound stayed closed. If the calendula treatment was stopped, the wound opened and the itch returned.

Allow deep wounds to heal inside before applying calendula; if the outer skin heals ahead of the deeper layers, you risk sealing in bacteria.

Taken internally, calendula treats a variety of mucosal troubles. Try it, for instance, for intestinal or bladder problems. A tea or tincture helps broken bones knit faster, too.

Calendula tea helps regulate menstruation. Drink two or three cups a day for a week before your period is due. This also helps prevent crampy menses. (For painful menses in general, though, check your intake of magnesium and vitamin B.)

Calendula is styptic—that is, it stops bleeding both internally and externally. (Obviously, for internal bleeding you should see a doctor as soon as possible!)

Use calendula internally as a tea or a tincture, and externally as an oil, a salve, a wrap, or a wash.

Don't use the green parts in teas. They *(hack)* can *(hack)* irritate *(hack)* the *(hack)* throat *(hack)*.

Calendula tea

2 teaspoons dried or fresh calendula flowers or petals
1 cup (250 ml) boiling water

Pour the boiling water over the herb. Steep for 10 minutes. Strain. Drink three cups a day, or let steep until the liquid is cool, and use externally for things such as skin cleansing.

Note: Again, tea made from steeping the green parts of calendula can irritate the throat.

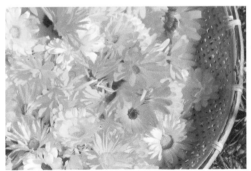

Bright yellow and orange calendula flowers.

Calendula tincture

From fresh flowers:

4 ounces (100 g) fresh flowers, either whole flower heads or just the petals
8 fluid ounces (1 cup) (200 ml) 95 % grain alcohol (190 proof)

From dried flowers:

4 ounces (100 g) dried flowers, either whole flower heads or just the petals
20 fluid ounces (2.5 cups) (500 ml) 50 % grain alcohol (100 proof)

Put the flowers or petals into a pint jar, cover with the alcohol, and close the lid tightly. Let steep for two to four weeks. Then strain, bottle, and label (example: "Dried Calendula, 1:5 50 %, 03.2021, purchased").

Dosage is 5 to 30 drops, one to four times a day.

Oil and salve of calendula

Make an herbal oil from the dried herb (page 18), and then make a salve from the oil (page 22).

It's good for wounds and for the skin in general.

Calendula butter salve

1 part fresh crushed calendula petals
1 part unsalted butter

Pour the ingredients into a small pan, mix, and heat the mixture until the butter is the color of the calendula. Strain. Store in the fridge—this will go rancid rather fast. Use as you would any calendula salve.

Calendula compress

1 ounce (30 g) fresh calendula
or 0.5 ounces (15 g) dried calendula
2 cups (500 ml) water

Add water and herb to a pan, bring to a boil, simmer for 5 minutes, and steep for 15 minutes longer. Strain and cool until just skin-comfortable. Dip a towel or rag in the tea, and squeeze out excess liquid. Put the moist, hot towel on the hurt spot and leave it there for 30–40 minutes.

Use for bruises, sprains, abrasions, wounds or tired eyes.

Always make a new tea for each application. This is especially important if you use the compress for your eyes or open wounds.

FOOD USES

The leaf is edible, but it's not all that tasty. It has about the same mineral content as dandelion leaf, so theoretically it makes sense to add calendula leaves to food.

You also can add fresh petals to salads and drinks, or as a garnish. Add the dried petals to soups, baked goods, and rice.

Calendula's bright orange petals have been used in place of saffron, but although it gives foods the same yellow color, calendula lacks saffron's flavor.

OTHER USES

A rinse with a strong calendula tea gives a golden tint to blond hair: Make 2 quarts (liters) strong calendula tea, strain (this is important!), and cool. Use it to rinse your hair, catching the leftovers in a bowl, and repeat at least 15 times. Finish by letting the tea dry in your hair.

WARNINGS

Calendula contains no sesquiterpene lactones. That means that it's not in the same allergenic league as mugwort or yarrow. It's still possible to get allergic reactions from calendula. This is, however, rare.

The plant's green parts, taken internally, can irritate mucous membranes in sensitive people.

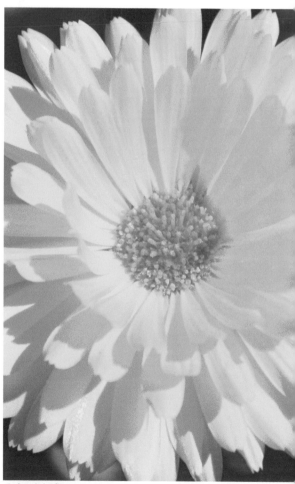

Calendula flower.

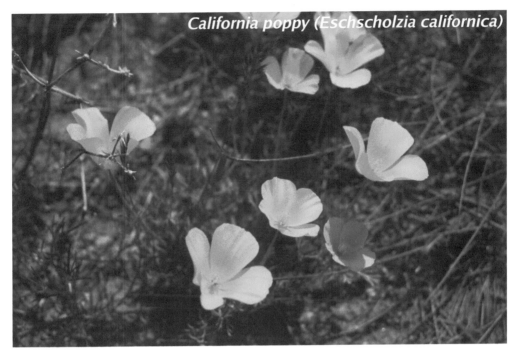
California poppy (Eschscholzia californica)

CALIFORNIA POPPY

A desert beauty that thrives in our gardens.

Eschscholzia californica: Also called gold poppy.

Family: Poppy family, *Papaveraceae*

Annual: Harvest in summer.

Habitat: California poppy comes from dry areas of California and Arizona.

Cultivation: It thrives in sandy soil in full sun. Sow the seeds straight outdoors. California poppy flowers throughout the summer. Its stalks can grow as tall as 36 inches (1 m). Although the branches are upright at first, they soon flop over anything growing downhill of the plant.

This poppy self-seeds profusely. The seeds can almost always survive our harsh winters, especially if the snowcover has been good. If you want to save some seeds, keep the poppy heads in a closed paper bag. The pods can explode and scatter their small round seeds everywhere.

Appearance: California poppy flowers are as much as 2 inches (4–5 cm) across; their color can be yellow, orange, white, or dark red. Leaves are gray green, clammy to the touch, and finely divided. The seedpods are 2–4 inches (5–10 cm) long. The taproot is around a quarter-inch (5 mm) in diameter, straight, an almost translucent orange brown, with a bright orange juice. The juice of the rest of the plant is colorless.

Look-alikes: None

Important constituents: Calming alkaloids, flavonoid

PICKING AND PROCESSING

In early summer the flowering plant is so pretty you won't want to pick it. But by late summer, when the stalks have grown too long and the flowers too few, it's easy to take a firm grip of the plant base and yank it up. Because the taproot is straight and thin, this is easy.

Remove dead and yellowed leaves, cut off the roots, and cut the remaining plant parts into 1-inch (2–3 cm) lengths.

If you want your plants to continue flowering, cut the aboveground parts a little above the soil. Leave a few leaves, and don't pull on the root.

EFFECTS AND USES

California poppy is an excellent herb for sleeplessness. It's almost specific for people who toss and turn, pondering the future, mulling over the day that was, or worrying about important life decisions—anyone whose head is so full of thoughts there's no room left for sleep.

It's also good for sleeplessness due to pain or discomfort.

Try a mix of California poppy with a tincture of either milky oats or St. John's wort.

I prefer tinctures for sleeplessness. You can keep the bottle ready at your bedside for early intervention, instead of grasping at sleep for hours before finally getting up to make some Sleepytime tea.

California poppy helps you sidestep stress. It's generally calming.

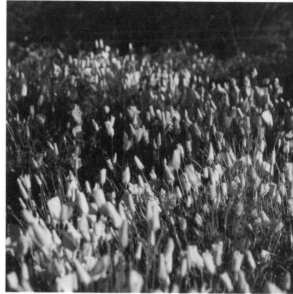

Sleepy 7 a.m. flowers of California poppy. Its Swedish common name is sömntuta, *"sleepyhead."*

If you take it during the day for tension, you may become sleepy at first, but a sense of alertness will return, and you'll feel calm and collected.

California poppy is good for pain, too, especially the normal pain that medication won't touch. Try this plant, too, if your pain causes you anxiety or depression.

Massage a few drops of diluted tincture into the gums of a teething baby. (I prefer chamomile for this, though: dip a cloth in chamomile tea, freeze it, and then give it to baby to chew on.)

Although California poppy contains alkaloids akin to those of its cousin the opium poppy, they're not addictive or "mindblowing." California poppy is therefore excellent for those trying to kick a dependence on opium alkaloid.

California poppy tincture

From fresh herb:

- 4 ounces (100 g) fresh herb, in 1/3–1-inch (1–3 cm) lengths
- 8 fluid ounces (200 ml) 190 proof grain alcohol (95 %)

From dried herb:

- 4 ounces (100 g) dried herb, in 1/3–1-inch (1–3 cm) lengths
- 20 fluid ounces (500 ml) 100 proof grain alcohol (50 %)

Put the herb pieces in a glass jar, cover with the alcohol, and close the lid tightly. Steep two to four weeks, strain and bottle. Label (example, fresh: "California poppy, 1:2 95 %, 6.2021, my garden"; example, dried: "California poppy, 1:5 50 %, 09.2021, Grandma's garden"). Dosage is 10 drops as needed. Repeat every 10 to 20 minutes, if necessary.

California poppy tea

- 1–2 teaspoons dried or fresh herb
- 1 cup (250 ml) boiling water

Pour boiling water over the herb, steep for 10 minutes, and strain. Drink a cup as needed, and take another cup within 30–60 minutes.

The tea is an acquired taste. I recommend the tincture.

OTHER USES

California poppy root makes bright-orange temporary tattoos. They'll last a few hours, and then rub off naturally, or you can rub them off right away with a damp rag if you want to try again.

WARNINGS

Don't use California poppy if you're pregnant. Some of its alkaloids have an oxytocic effect.

California poppy can show up as an opiate in some drug tests.

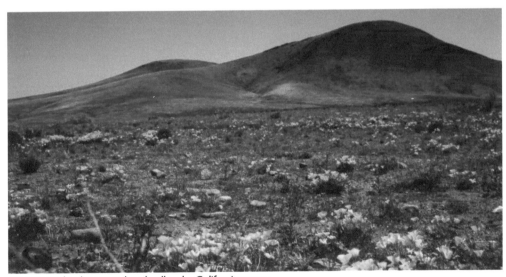

An Arizona landscape colored yellow by California poppy.

MALLOW-FAMILY MUCILAGINOUS PLANTS

Plants that contain mucilage soothe our mucous membranes (provided they don't also contain harsh acids or tannins).

The mallow family includes many such soothing plants. Try to include one in your remedies for inflammations—when our mucous membranes need soothing.

The mucilaginous mallows also nicely round out the flavor of many herbal tea blends.

Use the flowers and leaves of hollyhock (*Alcea rosea*); roots, flowers, and leaves of marshmallow (*Althaea officinalis*); leaves, flowers, and roots of true mallows (*Malva* species), tree mallows (*Lavatera* species), and globemallows (*Sphaeralcea* species).

You can even use the potted Chinese hibiscus in your living room (*Hibiscus rosa-sinensis*)—provided, of course, that you haven't sprayed it with anything toxic.

You can't use all parts of all mallow family plants, however. For instance, roselle (*Hibiscus sabdariffa*) is too sour to be soothing. And cotton root is too astringent.

But the usual gentle mallow family plants? Go for them!

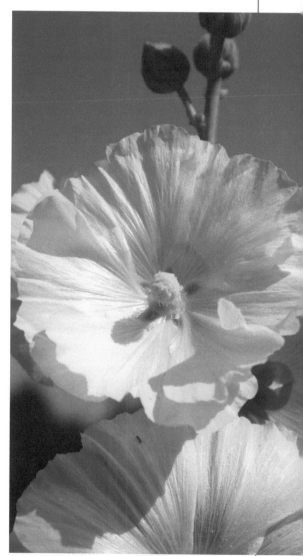

A white-flowered hollyhock (Alcea rosea*).*

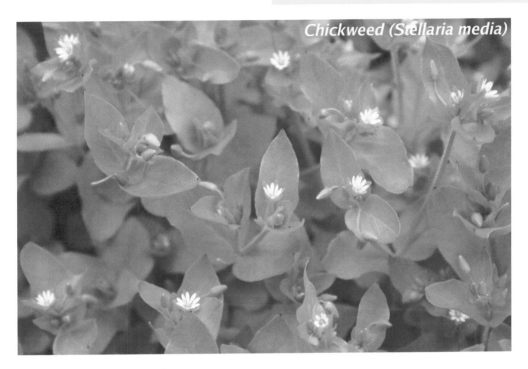
Chickweed (Stellaria media)

CHICKWEED

Hens love chickweed. Perhaps we should, too.

Stellaria media: Also called adder's mouth, chick wittles

Family: Pink family, *Caryophyllaceae*

Annual: Harvest from early summer to fall.

Habitat: Chickweed commonly grows in moist, rich soil, such as that of gardens and moist meadows. Its lush growth indicates that an area is suitable for cultivation.

You also may notice stunted plants growing along dry, sandy roads.

Cultivation: You won't need to encourage chickweed to grow in your yard or garden.

Appearance: Where chickweed thrives, it can grow into a dense groundcover as tall as 8 inches (20 cm). In such places, the nethermost leaves wither away (as will any smaller plants with the misfortune to have sprouted there first).

Chickweed stems are 2–20 inches (5 to 50 cm) long, much branched, and smooth but for a line of hairs along one side of each stem (this is sometimes absent on the flower stalks). The leaves are usually bald, but sometimes they'll be hairy at the base.

Look-alikes: You can't really confuse succulent chickweed with other plants, especially if it grows in a garden.

A few other species of *Stellaria* can look like chickweed, but they're differently haired. There are no toxic lookalikes (in Finland), but other species lack the effects and flavor of chickweed.

Important constituents: 4 ounces (100 g) dried chickweed contains 0.98 g potassium, 1.4 g calcium, 141 mcg chromium, 0.62 g magnesium, and 29.6 mg iron (Mark Pedersen, 1994); 4.8% potassium, 1.8% calcium, 2.9% magnesium, 7–12% mucilage 0.34% iron (James Duke, 1992). Chickweed's most important nutrient is vitamin C, with about 350 mg in 100 g dried herb.

Because chickweed is so rich in minerals and vitamins, it's a general strengthener and is suitable for long-term use.

PICKING AND PROCESSING

Harvest the aboveground parts. It will be easier to clean your take if you snip the herb with scissors instead of ripping it from the ground. Remove any yellow and dead parts and foreign plant matter.

Storing

Freezing. Cut the fresh herb in 1-inch (2–3 cm) lengths and freeze in small airtight bags or jars.

Or chop the fresh herb, add a little water, and freeze the mess in ice cube trays. Transfer the frozen cubes to airtight bags.

Juicing. Freeze the juice in airtight bags or ice cube trays. Or use alcohol: add one part in three of vodka, or one part in nine of 190 proof (95 percent) alcohol to your fresh juice (for example, 1 fluid ounce vodka to 3 fluid ounces fresh juice).

Infused oil. Make an herbal oil from the fresh or frozen herb (page 18). Use the oil immediately, or let the water settle out and make it into a salve (page 22).

Drying. Dry your chickweed, and then cut the dried herb into 1-inch (2–3 cm) lengths. Store the dried herb in airtight jars in a dark cupboard.

Chopping chickweed

I've tried to chop chickweed in a blender, but the fibrous stems wrapped themselves around the blades and choked the machine. My juicer didn't like the tough stems, either.

If your kitchen appliances can't cut chickweed, chop a quart (liter) of the herb with a sharp knife. Mix in cold water to make a slurry, and let the mix stand for a while. Use the resulting liquid right away, or freeze it.

EFFECTS AND USES

Fresh chickweed is ideal for relieving itches and treating inflamed skin. Use it externally in eczema, for wounds that just won't heal, or just to please your skin (for this, use fresh chopped chickweed or chickweed juice).

Use the herb externally and internally for psoriasis.

If your child itches all over with chickenpox, gently wash the skin with a cooled chickweed tea or a soothing chickweed ice cube several times a day.

Apply freshly squeezed chickweed juice straight on mosquito bites and similar itchinesses. It's easy. Just take a handful of lush chickweed, make it into a ball, and *sque-e-e-eze* it until a few drops of juice drip off your hand. Catch the drops and use them!

Other chickweed preparations work for mosquito bites, as well, from cooled tea to salve. Drink a tea from the fresh or dried herb to help with swellings and joint problems. The tea is also helpful in productive coughs.

Also use the herb internally for its vitamin C and mineral content.

Oil and salve of chickweed

Make an herbal oil from the fresh herb (page 18), and then make a salve from the oil (page 22). Apply to itchiness, rashes, and insect bites.

Chickweed tea

1–2 teaspoons dried or fresh chickweed
1 cup (250 ml) boiling water

Pour boiling water over the herb, steep for 10 minutes, and strain. Drink three to four cups a day.

Juiced chickweed

fresh chickweed

Cut older, fibrous chickweed into 1-inch (2–3 cm) lengths. Run the herb through the juicer.

Freeze the fresh juice to store it, or use it right away.

Chickweed syrup

1/2 cup (100 ml) juiced chickweed
or 1/2 cup (100 ml) liquid from chopped
  chickweed
1/2 cup sugar (100 ml)

Mix. Take a teaspoonful three times a day for a productive cough. (Or make a syrup; see page 27).

Chickweed-juice tea

1 tablespoon chickweed juice or liquid
1 cup (250 ml) boiled water

Pour the chickweed juice or liquid into the hot water. Drink.

FOOD USES

In any number of wild-food books you'll read that chickweed is a nice wild green, fresh or boiled, in all sorts of salty and meaty dishes. I've given it a try a few times. I find that if I eat it as a green (that is, in larger amounts than I would as a medicinal herb), my teeth get the same sort of unpleasant film I get from unripe bananas.

It's a good idea to cut the herb into half-inch (1 cm) pieces before you incorporate it into salads and boiled foods.

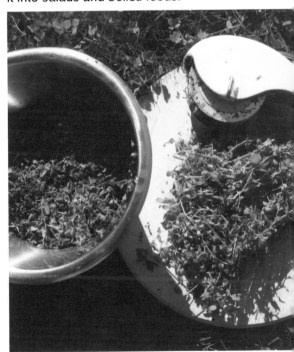

Hand-chopped fresh chickweed.

Chickweed stems are tough, and, given a chance and left long, they'll settle between teeth.

The best time to harvest chickweed for food is in early summer, before it flowers. If you use scissors to cut the crispy green tops, you'll avoid the tedious cleaning of yellow, dead, or moldy parts and soil. You'll also leave the tough older stems behind.

Butterfried chickweed

1 quart (liter) rinsed, cleaned chickweed tops
2–3 tablespoons butter
salt, lemon juice

Melt the butter in a pan, add the chickweed, and saute for 5 to 10 minutes. Add lemon juice and salt to taste, and serve.

A wild green smoothie

1–2 handfuls rinsed, cleaned greens (such as dandelion leaf, plantago leaf, chickweed, pennywort, willowherb, goutweed, lady's mantle)
2 cups (500 ml) buttermilk, yogurt, kefir, or the like
salt to taste

Cut the herbs in 1-inch (2–3 cm) lengths. Put them in the blender and whirl. Mix in the dairy.

Drink every day for a few weeks as a spring tonic.

Cheesy chickweed salad

1 quart (liter) rinsed, cleaned chickweed tops
4–8 ounces (100–200 g) grated cheese

Mix and serve with toast.

WARNINGS

Chickweed can contain nitrates. Don't give it to children younger than a year.

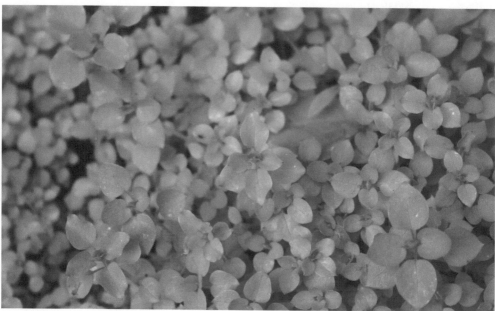

Young chickweed growth in spring.

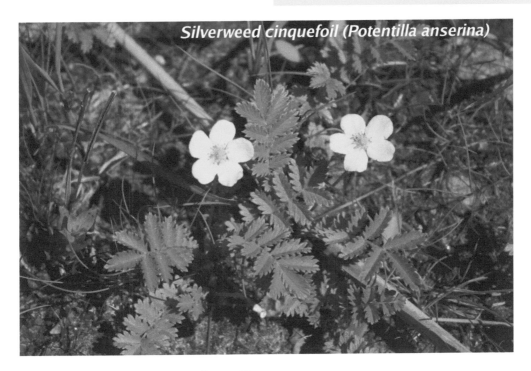

Silverweed cinquefoil (Potentilla anserina)

THE CINQUEFOILS

An herb to give you elbows, to bolster you against external pressures.

***Potentilla* species:** Including

- Silverweed cinquefoil (*Potentilla anserina*), a groundcover with rowan-like leaves. The yellow flowers are about a third to three-quarters of an inch (1-2 cm) across. The plant thrives in sand or gravel. The leaves get enormous if the plant is allowed into a flower bed. In sunny spots the runners are red; elsewhere they're green.

- Hoary cinquefoil (*Potentilla argentea*), an upright, grayish plant with yellow flowers about a third of an inch (1 cm) across. The leaves are usually three-, five- or sevenfingered. The plant likes dry meadows and ditches.

- Common tormentil (*Potentilla erecta*). An erect plant. The yellow flowers are about a third of an inch (1 cm) across; they usually have only four petals. It grows in moist sunny spots in deciduous forests.

- Marsh cinquefoil (*Potentilla palustris*). An upright swamp plant with reddish-brown flowers about an inch (2–3 cm) across. Very pretty in flower.

- Shrubby or bush cinquefoil (*Potentilla fruticosa*; also *Dasiphora fruticosa*). A bush. The yellow flowers are an inch (2–3 cm) across.

Family: Rose family (*Rosaceae*).

Perennial: Harvest from summer to fall.

Habitat: Most cinquefoils grow in dry and sunny places.

55

Cultivation: Bush cinquefoil is grown as an ornamental. It starts growing late in spring but is quite showy in fall. Because it looks like a well-used broom in spring and early summer, I replaced most of my bushes with various perennials.

None of the other cinquefoils require cultivation (in Finland); they arrive of their own accord.

Marsh cinquefoil does well transplanted to a garden pond.

Appearance: The leaves are lobed, except those of silverweed. The flowers have five petals, except for those of tormentil. The flowers are yellow, except for those of marsh cinquefoil. (There are many exotic species and cultivars in various shades of orange and red, or even white.) The plants are herbaceous, except for bush cinquefoil.

Look-alikes: It's possible to confuse the normal yellow-flowered lobed-leafed cinquefoil with buttercups, which have similar lobed leaves and yellow flowers. But the surfaces of cinquefoil flowers are always matte, and those of buttercups always shiny.

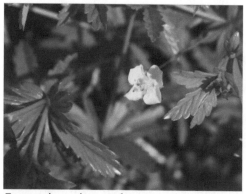

Four petals are the norm for common tormentil flowers.

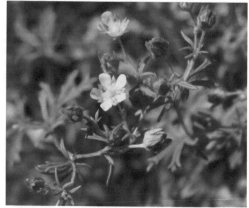

Hoary cinquefoil (Potentilla argentea): deeply divided leaves, five petals. Most cinquefoils follow this pattern.

Don't pick "cinquefoils" with shiny flowers. Buttercups irritate mucous membranes and skin. Some species of buttercup are so irritating they produce long-lasting sores (but these look nothing like cinquefoils).

Important constituents: Tannins, glycosides, bitters, flavonoids (cinquefoil leaves); up to 25 % tannins, red pigment, small amounts of volatile oil (tormentil root)

PICKING AND PROCESSING

Gather the leaf or the flowering tops in summer or fall. Spread your harvest indoors out of the light on old cotton bedsheets or the like, spread on layer of newspapers. You can also dry the herb in hanging bundles.

Store in airtight glass jars.

Years-old herb that has lost most of its color has also lost most of its effect. Pick new cinquefoils at least as often as every two or three years.

You can use the leaves and flowering tops of common tormentil as you would any other cinquefoil, but digging its roots is hard, slow work. The roots are small, about the size of the last joint of a little finger.

Alternatively, alder cones (*Alnus* species) give the same effect of protecting the gut lining in severe intestinal inflammation, and picking alder cones is a wonderful experience: you get to start your herb-harvesting in the middle of winter, when everything is covered in snow.

If you wash and slice the fresh root of a common tormentil, the yellowish-gray cut surface will develop a reddish tinge. If you cut an alder, the cut surface will turn deep red. The Finnish name for alder reflects this: *leppä* is an old word for blood.

If you absolutely must dig up tormentil roots, rinse them and cut them in 1/6-inch (5 mm) slices. Spread them to dry, or use

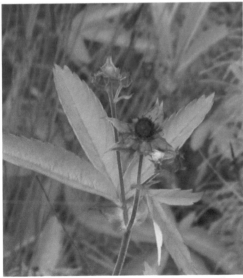

*The dark red flower of marsh cinquefoil (*Potentilla palustris*).*

a dehydrator. Dried roots are not as strong as fresh ones.

The roots of ground-covering cinquefoils have been used as astringents and their runners for survival food.

EFFECTS AND USES

Cinquefoils help you defend yourself. They grow you elbows, and give even a doormat the strength to say "no."

The overstressed person gets great help from cinquefoils. After you've eaten the leaves for a month or two, you notice that you don't have to keep two boyfriends, three jobs, and five hobbies. Suddenly you have time for the things that really are important to you—and no stress.

Cinquefoils shield you from external influences. You no longer care what anyone else thinks you should or should not do. You can follow your own way. It's enough to eat one leaf (about the size of a one-euro coin or U.S. "silver dollar") every day, or to add cinquefoil to your daily herbal tea.

Cinquefoils relieve menstrual and gut cramps, especially in those who suffer without complaining.

(Those who complain without suffering find chamomile excellent, instead.) Sip the tea or eat a leaf every 10 minutes until the pain stops, usually within half an hour. Also, if you are subject to menstrual cramps, increase your dietary magnesium intake.

Cinquefoils are typical rose-family astringents.

Astringent herbs tighten swollen membranes and so help relieve inflammations locally.

Drink a tea of cinquefoil for mild diarrhea, gargle for inflamed mouth and throat mucosa, wash small wounds with it, or dab some cooled tea onto sunburned skin.

Note that you can substitute agrimony (*Agrimonia* species), both for the elbows and for the astringent effect.

Refer to page 96 for more information about rose family astringents.

Cinquefoil tea

1–2 teaspoons dried or fresh cinquefoil
 leaves or flowering tops
1 cup (250 ml) boiling water

Pour water over the herb, steep for 10 minutes, and strain.

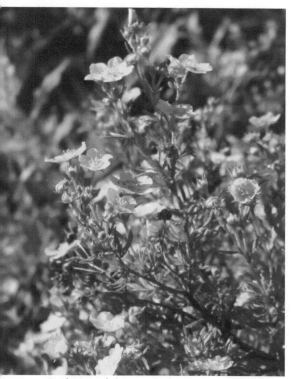

*Bush cinquefoil (*Potentilla fruticosa*) in flower.*

Cinquefoil paste

1–2 teaspoons powdered cinquefoil leaf
1 egg yolk

Mix. Apply to inflamed cuticles. Leave the paste on for 30 minutes. Wash off with mild soap.

Tormentil root decoction

1–2 teaspoons dried sliced roots of tormentil
1 cup (250 ml) cold water

Add the herb and water to a pan, bring to a boil, let boil for 10 minutes, and strain.

Drink up to three cups a day in small sips for diarrhoea or similar gut problems.

Strong tormentil root decoction

3 teaspoons dried sliced roots of tormentil
1 cup (250 ml) cold water

Add the herb and the water to apan, bring to a boil, let boil for 10 minutes, cool, and strain.

Use externally to wash small wounds, hemorrhoids, frostbite, abrasions, or sunburned skin.

FOOD USES

Add cinquefoil leaves or flowers to salads, soups, stews, and herbed spreads.

WARNINGS

Because the tannins in tormentil root can irritate the gut, never drink more than three cups of the tea in a day.

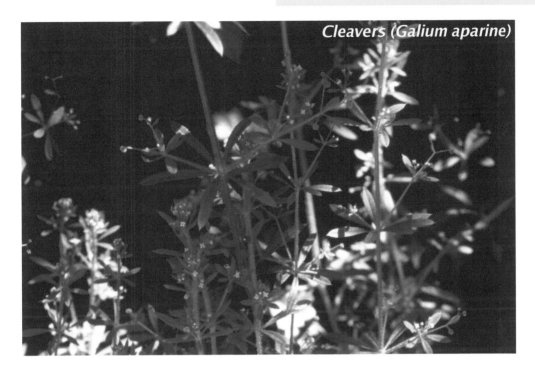

Cleavers (Galium aparine)

CLEAVERS

Cleavers will stick to anything. Lady's bedstraw has a pleasant scent.

Galium species: Including
- Lady's bedstraw (*Galium verum*); other names: yellow spring bedstraw, cheese rennet, yellow bedstraw
- Cleavers (*Galium aparine*); other names: stickywilly, catchweed, goosegrass
- False cleavers (*Galium spurium*; *Galium aparine* var. *spurium*)

Family: Madder family, *Rubiaceae*

Annual/perennial: The two cleavers species are annuals; lady's bedstraw is perennial. Harvest in summer.

Habitat: Cleavers like damp rich soil. Lady's bedstraw grows on dry sunny meadows or roadsides.

Appearance: Cleavers have long stems with tiny hooks on every stem, leaf, and seed that stick easily to dog's fur and your woollen socks or sweater. The seeds are tiny, round, green, and paired. The white flowers are tiny.

Lady's bedstraw can become almost a shrub—some branches are woody by the end of summer—but it does die back every winter. The flowers are small, but the mass of them makes for showy flower stalks. They are nicely scented. Leaves are dark green and needle-like.

A hybrid with white bedstraw (*Galium album*) is paler yellow and unscented.

Look-alikes: The other bedstraws are look-alikes, but I haven't used them. The aforementioned species have a long history of use and are sufficiently abundant not to stray from.

Bedstraws are nontoxic.

Important constituents: Silica, plant acids, vitamin C (lady's bedstraw); glycosides, plant acids, flavonoids (cleavers)

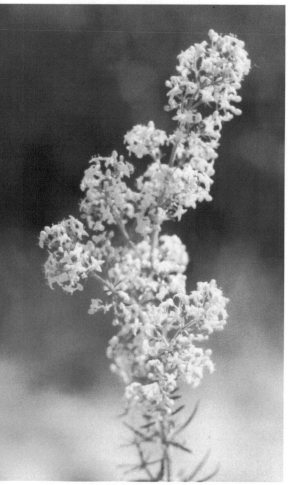

Flowers of lady's bedstraw (Galium verum).

PICKING AND PROCESSING

For lady's bedstraw, cut the flower stalks above the woody part. Take at most a fifth of any given plant. If the plant under your hand has but three flower stalks, let it grow, and find a larger plant to harvest from.

For cleavers, pull the green stalks off the tall grass or from among the vegetables where they grow. Remove any brown and black parts and foreign matter.

Cut bedstraws into 1-inch (2–3 cm) pieces and spread them on a cloth to dry indoors out of the light.

You can also make small bundles of lady's bedstraw stalks and hang them to dry. Cleavers can be hung to dry, too: just drape it over a piece of string and press the parts together lightly to make it stick to itself.

If the season has been wet, you can juice cleavers in a juicer. Cut the stalks up first. Freeze the juice in ice cube trays or use immediately. Store the cubes in airtight freezer containers or bags.

EFFECTS AND USES

The bedstraws are lymphatics; they help with inflamed lymph nodes, with scar tissue, with slowly healing wounds and sores, with eczema, and with cysts. They can also be of help in some joint troubles.

The bedstraws are fairly good for treating some benign tumors, such as fibroids. Drink three or four cups of cleavers tea a day. If the benign tumor is on the skin, cool the herb used to make the tea slightly and apply it like a poultice.

Bedstraws are cooling, so you can use them to take down a high fever.

And because the bedstraws are also mildly diuretic, anti-inflammatory, and astringent, they're useful for treating urinary tract infections. For urinary gravel and sand, combine bedstraw with mallow leaf or root, or with other mucilaginous herbs, such as psyllium seed.

Take bedstraw tea when you're recuperating from a bad flu, an operation, or a broken bone; it's rich in minerals.

People prone to psoriasis benefit from drinking up to three cups of the tea every day for a few months. Psoriasis sufferers should also look into their vitamin D levels.

Juice from a crushed wad of fresh cleavers can be applied straight for various skin problems and insect bites.

Cleavers tea

1–2 teaspoons dried cleavers
1 cup (250 ml) boiling water

Pour water over the herb, steep for 10 minutes, and strain. Drink up to three cups a day.

Cleavers maceration

4–5 tablespoons dried herb
3 cups (750 ml) cold water

Pour water into a jar, add the herb, steep 4–12 hours, and strain. Drink up to three cups a day.

Juiced cleavers

fresh cleavers, cut in 1-inch (2–3 cm) pieces

Add cleavers to your blender with a little water. Blend and strain.

Mix 2–3 tablespoons cleavers juice into 8 ounces (250 ml) cold water and drink up to three cups a day.

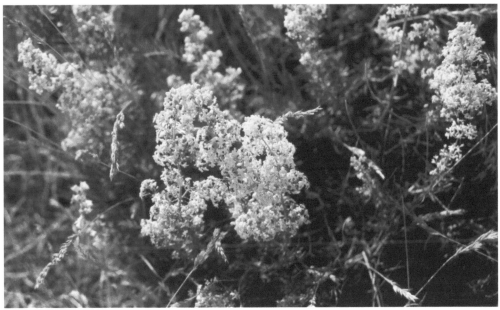

Lady's bedstraw (Galium verum).

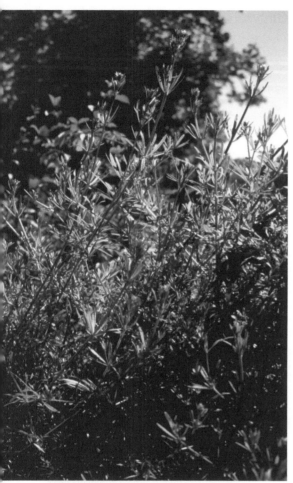

FOOD USES

A strong decoction of lady's bedstraw, or the fresh juice of cleavers, work as rennet in warm milk.

You can make a coffee-like drink from roasted cleavers seed: harvest the seeds, dry them, and shake them around in a bag with some small stones to get rid of the hooks. Now rinse the seeds, drain excess water, and roast them in a cast-iron pan. Grind and use as you would coffee beans. The resulting beverage has a scent of coffee (but not the flavor).

OTHER USES

Roots of lady's bedstraw makes the same red color you get from madder root (*Rubia tinctorum*).

But lady's bedstraw is a wildflower on the decline, and it takes 2 pounds (1 kg) of the dried root to color 4 ounces (100 grams) of wool.

A lush rush of cleavers striving for the sky.

A cleavers beverage

This recipe is from the 1861 translation of the 1230 book *Meddygedon Myddfai* (The Physicians of Myddvai):

Take the whole herb, leaves, blossoms, and seed included, (as the season may be), and pound them together well: then put in an unglazed earthenware vessel, and fill it up without pressing them; then pour thereon as much as it will admit of pure spring water, and let it stand a night.

Some say that it is best that a quarter of it should be sea water, or water salted as much as sea water, for the first week of drinking; then ceasing from the salt water, it should be taken fresh as the only drink for nine weeks.

It is wonderful how strong and healthy you will become in that time.

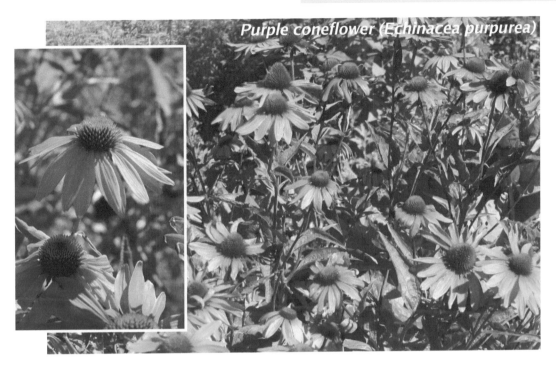

Purple coneflower (Echinacea purpurea)

THE CONEFLOWERS

Garden beauties for the immune system.

Echinacea species:
- Purple coneflower (*Echinacea purpurea*); common names include Eastern purple coneflower, black sampson, red sunflower
- Narrowleaf coneflower (*Echinacea angustifolia*); common names include black sampson, Kansas snakeroot
- Pale purple coneflower (*Echinacea pallida*); common names include pale coneflower, pale echinacea

Family: Daisy family, *Asteraceae* (*Compositae*: *Tubuliflorae*)

Perennial: Harvest green parts and flowers in summer, roots and seeds in autumn.

Habitat: Coneflowers come from the tall-grass prairies of North America. The grass keeps them rather smaller than garden specimens.

Cultivation: Purple coneflower is easy to grow: sow the seeds, add some fertilizer and lime, and keep the small plants free from weeds.

The other coneflowers are more demanding, their germination rate isn't as good, and the plants usually succumb to harsh winters.

As with other perennials, you'll get only a few leaves during the first summer. In the second summer, one or two flowers appear. After that, a well-tended plant flowers abundantly each summer.

The American prairies are chalky. Your garden coneflowers will thrive if the soil is pH 7–8; they'll also be at their strongest as medicinal plants.

A sunny spot, and lime added to acid soil, will reward you with dozens of flowers.

Appearance: Purple coneflower (*Echinacea purpurea*) grows to about 36 inches (1 m) with light purple flowers from 3 to 4 inches (7–10 cm) across. Cultivars can have larger flowers colored dark purple to white. They all work. This species doesn't have carrot-like taproots.

Narrowleaf coneflower (*Echinacea angustifolia*) is smaller in size, with smaller, more compact flowers. This species has a taproot.

Pale purple coneflower (*Echinacea pallida*) is taller. Its flower petals are long and flimsy; they'll blow on the breeze or hang straight down. This species has a taproot.

Look-alikes: You might find similarly large purple flowers, but they don't usually sport the spiky round seedhead.

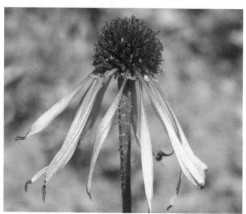

The flower of pale purple coneflower (Echinacea pallida).

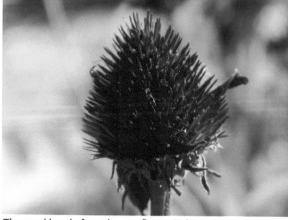

The seed head of purple coneflower (Echinacea purpurea).

Important constituents: Alcamides (isobutylamides, etc.), caffeic acid derivatives (phenols, phenol propanes, cichoric acid, echinacosides, etc.), flavonoids, polysaccharides (arabinogalactan, etc.), and a trace of essential oils (sesquiterpenes)

Alcamides dissolve well in strong alcohol. Polysaccharides dissolve in water. The caffeic-acid derivatives dissolve in both water and alcohol.

Roots of taprooted species of *Echinacea* contain as much as 20 percent inulin, a sugar that helps our digestive bacteria. It has nothing to do with insulin, which is a hormone we need to get blood sugar into our cells.

Isobutylamides account for the plant's "tingly-tongue" effect. Although the strength of the tingle tells something about the strength of a tincture, the poly-saccharides and caffeic acid derivatives also play roles in strengthening the immune system.

PICKING AND PROCESSING

Cut a third of the flower stalks in early fall and pick all the flowers.

Pick seed heads from remaining stalks in late fall, or dig the roots in fall or spring.

To prepare flowers to use in your wintery herbal teas, cut them into quarter-inch (5 mm) slices and spread them to dry. The flower's most important part is the white mass in the middle: it will numb your tongue briefly on contact.

Pick the seeds when they're ripe—that is, when the stalk has turned brown under the seed head. Cut the stalks and take the seed heads indoors to dry. Don some heavy leather gloves, and crush the dried seed heads.

Coneflower seed is light-brown or gray, square, and varies in size depending on species and growing conditions, from 1/8-inch to around 1/4-inch (5 mm) long, and at most 1/16-inch (1–2 mm) in diameter. The seeds have the same tongue-numbing (tingly) property of the flower's white mass. The rest of the seed head consists mostly of sharp spines. The botanical name (*Echinacea*) is a tribute to that: its prefix *echino-* is Greek for "spiny."

Dried coneflower stems and leaves aren't as strong as the flowers and seeds.

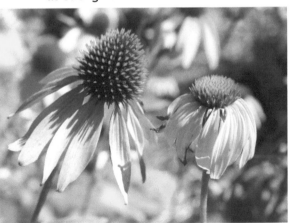

Flowers of purple coneflower—one with almost-ripe seeds, the other new and flat.

The roots of purple coneflower are small, and if you dig up the plant you won't be able to enjoy its showy flowers in the years to come. Use the roots of taprooted species, instead, if you can grow them.

EFFECTS AND USES

You can use any *Echinacea* species as medicine: they all work. You can use the roots or the aboveground parts: they all work. You can use them as teas, tinctures, powders, chewed, and as compresses—they all work.

Carry a bottle of tincture with you in flu season and take a few drops at the first signs of flu. (You could also use hot black currant juice or a hot tea with garlic, lemon juice, and honey, but those aren't as easy to carry in a handbag or rucksack.)

Take any coneflower as a tea or tincture when you have a full-blown flu, too. It helps keep opportunistic infections at bay and the immune system working on the virus.

Research indicates that coneflower enhances the mobility and efficacy of white blood cells.

Heating herbs, such as garlic, cayenne, and ginger, taken with *Echinacea* help move the waste products of viral war onward and out, thus lessening symptoms.

Use coneflowers as a tea or tincture externally and internally for small wounds, sprains, abrasions, contusions, and bruises.

Apply a coneflower tea to hemorrhoids (a tincture there would be a tad extreme).

Put three to five drops of tincture on wasp stings and take 15 drops every 10 minutes internally. The swelling will go down to the size of a mosquito-bite within an hour, and the ache and itch will disappear.

In the U.S., *Echinacea* tincture has been used for the more toxic stings and bites of scorpions, rattlesnakes, spiders, and the like. See a doctor as soon as possible, but until you get there, take large amounts—up to 2 fluid ounces (60 ml)—of *Echinacea* tincture at 10- to 30-minute intervals (and apply the tincture or tea externally). Reduce the amount and frequency of tincture only once the swelling subsides.

For skin problems caused by multiresistant *Staphylococcus aureus* (MRSA), pour a strong strained *Echinacea* tea over the affected area, and take the tincture internally. Also take one to three crushed raw garlic cloves before food at least once a day. Add a calendula tea internally and externally to the protocol, and—if you can find it—a

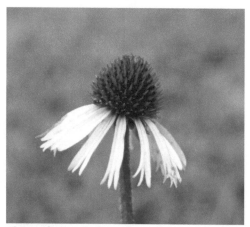

Flower of narrowleaf coneflower (Echinacea angustifolia).

tea, tincture, or syrup of elecampane (*Inula helenium*).

Coneflower remedies are generally more effective if you take small amounts often, rather than large amounts a few times a day. Three to ten drops every 10–30 minutes is better than 30–60 drops one to three times a day.

I don't recommend long-term intensive use of *Echinacea*.

I also think you shouldn't take out all mild respiratory tract infections the minute they appear. Our immune systems need a good workout every now and then. You'll be better prepared for worse problems if you let a mild infection get you every few years.

Use tingly preparations of coneflowers (or chew the seeds, the white mass inside the flowers, or the taproots) if you feel coneflower isn't helping your immune system. The isobutylamides raise body temperature and are more effective in so-called "cold" people.

The pyrrolizidine alkaloids in *Echinacea* species are nontoxic.

Tincture of Echinacea

From the fresh plant:

4 ounces (100 g) fresh greens, seeds, or roots of any *Echinacea*
8 fluid ounces (200 ml) 190 proof grain alcohol (95 %)

From the dried plant:

4 ounces (100 g) dried greens, seeds, or roots of any *Echinacea*
20 fluid ounces (2 cups, or 500 ml) 120 proof grain alcohol (60 %)

Put the herb in a glass jar, cover with the alcohol, and close the lid tightly. Steep two to four weeks.

Strain, bottle, and label (example, fresh plant: "Purple coneflower, 1:2 95 %, 08.2021, my garden"; example, dried plant: "*Echinacea pallida*, 1:5 60 %, 04.2021, storebought").

Take 15–100 drops up to five times a day, or from three to ten drops every 10–30 minutes.

Purple coneflower tea

1–2 teaspoons purple coneflower, fresh or dried
1 cup (250 ml) boiling water

Pour boiling water over the herb, steep for 10 minutes, and strain.

Drink up to five cups a day.

OTHER USES

Use the dried seed heads in dried flower arrangements. They'll retain their seeds if you dry them while the stem is green; do remove the petals, though. If you wait until the seeds are ripe and carefully strip the seeds, petals, and spines, you get a hatlike light-brown form for your dried flowers.

WARNINGS

Coneflowers aren't toxic, but if you have a complicated autoimmune disease, such as ulcerative colitis or Crohn's disease, be careful with the *Echinacea*. It may be totally benign for you, but it might also cause a flare-up of symptoms.

If you're allergic to mugwort, yarrow, or ragweed, you might get allergic symptoms from the aboveground parts of *Echinacea*. You may be able to take preparations made from the roots without problems.

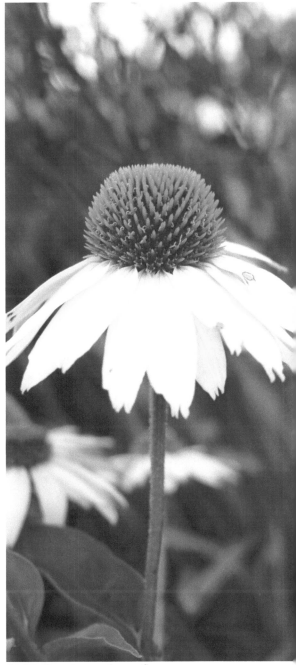

A white-flowering purple coneflower.

ADVICE FOR FLU SEASON

The following tips will get you through flu season relatively unscathed:

- Strengthen your overall health. Eat a varied diet rich in nutrients, avoid stress, get enough sleep, and exercise adequately.

- Wash your hands using water and (real) soap before you touch your mucous membranes. You can get viruses from touching money and door handles, among other things. A healthy immune system can repel them, but that becomes more difficult if you carry them straight to your mucous membranes.

- Avoid sugar. Reject candy, chocolates, and soft drinks, and, given a choice, pick something salty instead of a sweet pastry.

- If you get the flu, anyway, drink a lot of warm or hot fluids, and rest as much as you can. Good things to drink include hot juice of black currant or black elder (add only enough sugar to make the juice drinkable) and a tea made with garlic, lemon juice, and honey. (Those with reflux should avoid the garlic, though.)

- Don't get up to get things done too early after recovering from flu, or you may get a really bad bacterial infection. They take advantage of a weakened body and an overworked immune system. Don't start to exercise too early, either; that can bring on myocarditis.

- Avoid NSAIDs, such as acetyl salicylic acid (aspirin), ibuprofen (such as Advil), and acetaminophen (Tylenol and its ilk). These drugs can hamper the immune system, and that leads to more viruses in the cells and symptoms that hang on longer.

- Avoid flu medications. Or, if you do take them, understand what they do to you: because they usually contain caffeine, you won't notice when you're too tired to stay upright; because they contain painkillers, your achy muscles and head won't urge you to bed; because they dry up your mucous membranes, you won't have a runny nose to help your body quickly get rid of metabolic wastes—and they won't just dry up the nose, but all the body's mucosa. If you must take such medicines, remember: you are still ill. Don't do too much too fast, or the flu will simmer on low for a while and then bounce right back at you.

A garlic tea with lemon juice and honey

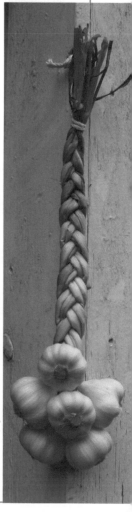

1 clove garlic, sliced
1 teaspoon honey
1 teaspoon lemon juice
1 cup (250 ml) boiling water

Put all ingredients in a cup and stir. Drink as soon as it's cooled enough to do so.

Make another cup right away. This is both tasty and healthful.

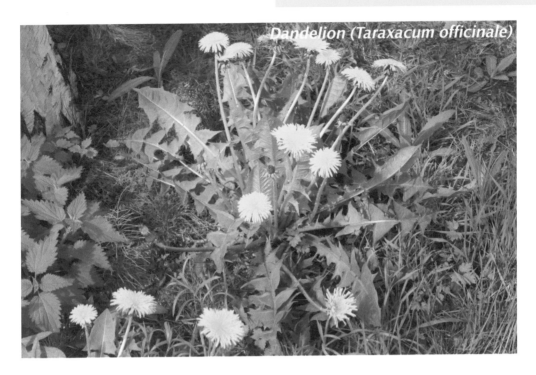
Dandelion (Taraxacum officinale)

DANDELION

Dandelion leaf is so diuretic, its French name is pissenlit—*"pee in bed."*

Taraxacum* species:** Also called lion's tooth. Officially, there are hundreds of dandelion species in Finland. A sane person calls the lot "dandelion," or ***Taraxacum officinale in botanical Latin.

Family: Daisy family (*Asteraceae*) (*Compositae: Liguliflorae*)

Perennial: Harvest in early summer (flowers), summer (leaves), or fall and spring (roots).

Habitat: Dandelion likes sunny spots, meadows, ditches, lawns, gravel, and sand.

Cultivation: Yes, dandelion seeds are sold by large seed companies. You can, if you wish, buy them and plant your garden in dandelions. Cultivars are usually selected for broader leaves or milder taste, but now and then you get bog-standard dandelions from such seeds.

In my garden, dandelion volunteers everywhere.

For easier digging at fall harvest, weed around your dandelions in summer.

Appearance: The flower stem is hollow, leafless, and supports only one flower. The basal leaves grow from a more-or-less carrot-shaped taproot. The white sap of dandelion makes an indelible impression on clothing, sparing neither summer dresses nor blue jeans. The sap turns brownish on skin overnight, but that's easily rubbed off.

Look-alikes: Legion. Here are a few.

Annual sowthistles (*Sonchus* species) sport many leaves and flowers on each flower stalk. Although they can be used as food greens, they aren't useful medicinally.

"Fall dandelion" or fall hawkbit (*Leontodon autumnalis*) lacks the hollow flower stem. It, too, is edible.

To the uninitiated, the large fluffballs of various goat's beards (*Tragopogon* species) may resemble dandelion puffs, but a closer look reveals differences, as does the growth habit. The greens of goat's beard, and especially their roots, have been used as wild foods. They have a mild taste. The plant is biennial, which means that roots dug from under flowering plants are too old. Locate and dig under nearby leaf rosettes, instead. Goat's beard is a wild cousin of salsify, a root vegetable. If you pick a goat's beard fluffball just before it opens completely and then carefully dry it, you'll have a very nice dried flower.

In early summer, coltsfoot (*Tussilago farfara*) can be mistaken for dandelion, but the yellow flowers of coltsfoot appear before the leaves, and the flower stalk has many small scales or leaflets. Although coltsfoot has been used as a wild green and herb, it contains liver-toxic pyrrolizidine alkaloids, and such use should be discontinued.

Important constituents: Bitters, minerals (potassium and others), vitamins A, B, C, flavonoids (leaf); bitters, inulin (as much as 40 % in fall, only 1–5 % in spring) (root).

Inulin is a sugar that helpful intestinal bacteria relish. Llarge amounts can cause bloating and gas.

PICKING AND PROCESSING

Harvest spring and summer dandelion leaves to use in salads.

Harvest its flowers of early summer to make a syrup or oil (and salve) from them.

Dandelion roots are at their sweetest in autumn. A other times of year they're either rather bitter or frozen. Dig the roots while the ground is frozen and wash them with a stiff brush. You needn't remove the bark; just clean them of small stones and earthworms. Cut the roots in pieces a quarter-inch (0.5 cm) thick by 2 inches (5 cm) long (or in quarter-inch slices), and dry them.

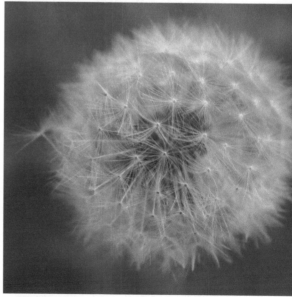

A dandelion puff.

EFFECTS AND USES

Don't take dandelion if you have low blood pressure. (See "Warnings," page 76).

Do take dandelion if your liver is stressed. Dandelion is outstanding for those with hepatitis or who work with solvents (such as alcohol, strong glue, strong cleaning agents, gasoline, paints, and essential oils). Professions that involve solvents include hairdresser, cleaner, furniture maker, car mechanic, painter, and aromatherapist. (Of course, the liver of an alcoholic also has been damaged by a solvent.)

The best way to take dandelion is to eat a matchstick-sized piece of the dried or fresh root three times a day, and to eat dandelion leaf salads three to seven times a week (while the leaf is available).

Dandelion's bitter taste aids digestion as follows:

• Its taste on the tongue makes saliva flow.
• This increases the secretions of the esophagus.
• And this increases stomach secretions,
• which increase bile secretion and secretions of the pancreas.
• And they increase secretions of the intestines.

All herbs and foods with a bitter taste work similarly, from chewed juniper berries (*Juniperus communis*), grapefruit juice, and various gentians (*Gentiana* species) to hops (*Humulus* species) and even Campari.

The strongest bitters lower blood sugar, so try to eat within half an hour of taking a strong bitter.

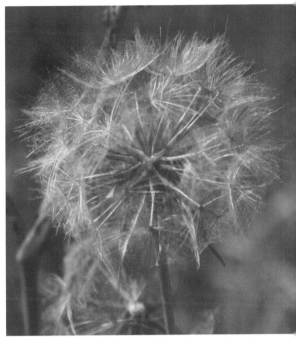

*The fluffball of goat's beard (*Tragopogon pratensis*).*

Use bitters such as dandelion to treat loss of appetite, heartburn from too little stomach acid, and other such problems stemming from a lowered digestive fire. If you feel like you're allergic to yet another food every other week, you may have an underactive digestion, and bitters help.

Also, cold foods cool an underactive digestion even further, so if you *must* eat salads or ice cream or drink sodas, heat them first and ingest them *warm*.

Finally, be liberal with warming spices. Follow these steps and in a week or two you'll notice your digestive troubles have lessened considerably, and you can again eat those formerly troublesome foods.

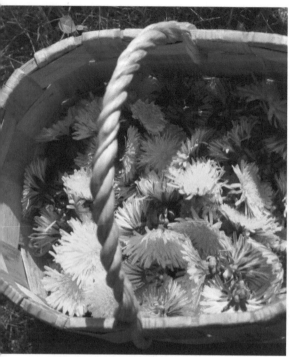
A basket of dandelion flowers.

Although dandelion (like burdock and similar strong herbal diuretics) can be used purely for its diuretic action, I believe in finding the cause of your swollen extremities and treating that. Strengthen the heart, the liver, the kidneys. If that approach doesn't help, it's a very good idea to see your doctor.

Because pharmaceutical diuretics usually leach potassium from the body, herbalists' cavalier use of strong diuretics can make an allopathic doctor gasp. But herbal diuretics such as dandelion, chicory, horsetail, burdock, and couchgrass all contain potassium. If in doubt, eat bananas or tomatoes with your diuretic herbs. They contain potassium, too.

The leaf of both dandelion and burdock can be found at the top of the "diuretic index." This is easy to demonstrate: give the tea to everyone who comes through the door, and then count how many must leave during your 90-minute lecture. The percent calculated from that is the diuretic index. Try it with different herbs (birch leaf and goldenrod are diuretics, too). Then reward your students with some peppermint tea, which is not diuretic.

Because of this diuretic activity, avoid taking a dandelion tea or eating a dandelion salad in the evening, or you may just find out why the French call dandelion *pissenlit*, "pee-a-bed."

The medicinal properties of chicory (*Cichorium intybus*) are equivalent to dandelion's. The root is less strong, but it's a lot larger: digging chicory is much easier than digging dandelion.

If you're really lazy, you can get dandelion (or chicory) roots without digging. Check herbal coffees for chicory (or dandelion) root content, and buy the brand that contains the most. Or buy endive, which is actually chicory greens, and use it as you would dandelion greens.

Dandelion also makes a wonderfully relaxing oil and salve.

Dandelion leaf tea

2–3 teaspoons young fresh dandelion leaves
1 cup (250 ml) boiling water

Pour boiling water over the herb, steep for 10 minutes, and strain.

Drink two to three cups a day.

Dandelion decoction

2 teaspoons dried leaf or root
1 cup (250 ml) cold water

Add the herb and water to a pan, bring to a boil, turn off heat, cover, and steep for 12 to 15 minutes. Strain and drink two to three cups a day.

Oil and salve of dandelion

Make an herbal oil from the fresh flowers (page 18), and then make a salve from the oil (page 22).

Apply for muscle, neck, and back pain; it's ideal for relaxing muscles tightened by emotions.

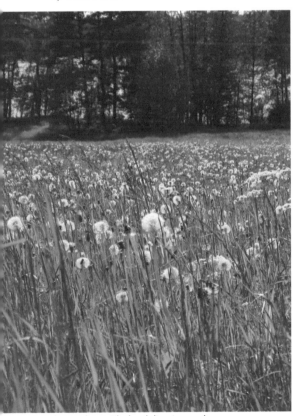

A meadow with dandelion in seed.

FOOD USES

Don't take dandelion if you have low blood pressure. (See "Warnings," page 76.)

Dandelion is best used in salads.

Although a dandelion salad can taste all too bitter at first, you'll get used to it if you start by eating small amounts daily. After a while you'll start to crave the bitter taste. After that you'll find the fried pieces of root or flower buds with croutons very tasty. You'll also love flower buds or flowers in omelets, stews, and soups.

Dandelion roots are sweetest if they're dug in the fall. Wash them, slice them, and fry them with onions and/or potatoes.

Less bitter leaves

These tips and tricks can lessen the bitterness of dandelion leaves:

- Cover the plants for a week before harvest.
- First simmer the leaves for 2 or 3 minutes in water with a little salt, and then pour off the liquid.
- Mix dandelion leaves with something else—for instance, willowherb leaf, boiled nettles, or potato mash.
- Soak the leaves in cold water for a few hours.
- Pick less deeply divided leaves.
- Remove each leaf's center vein (the bitterest part).

Dandelion syrup

Make a syrup using the recipe on page 27. Use whole dandelion flowers (no need to remove the green parts).

The small black beetles you often find on dandelion flowers will take off if you leave your harvest in the shade for an hour.

Dandelion syrup tastes a little of nuts and vanilla. If you leave some in the fridge to age, as years pass it will become more and more honey-like in flavor and consistency.

Dandelion salad

2–4 ounces (50–100 g) fresh dandelion leaves
2–4 ounces (50–100 g) leaves of other wild greens, such as goutweed, lady's mantle, black currant, birch, and/or willowherb
one or more of these ingredients:
2–4 ounces (50–100 g) lettuce
sliced boiled eggs
cubed feta cheese
cubed ripe tomatoes
olives
cubed boiled potatoes

Combine and add your favorite dressing, or try one of the following recipes.

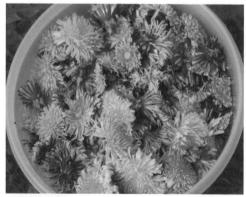

Dandelion flowers.

Dressings

Combine ingredients, then let your dressing mellow before mixing into the salad.

Sour cream

1–2 tablespoons orange juice
1 cup (250 ml) sour cream
1/4 teaspoon salt

Yogurt

2 tablespoons olive oil
2 tablespoons apple cider vinegar
2–3 tablespoons lowfat yogurt
pinch sugar
1/4 teaspoon salt
white pepper
chives

Mustard

1 tablespoon mustard
1–2 tablespoons apple cider vinegar
1–2 tablespoons olive oil
pinch sugar
pinch salt
white pepper

Grandma's special

1/2 cup (125 ml) mild-tasting oil
1/2 cup (125 ml) soy sauce or tamari
2–3 teaspoons sugar or honey
1 teaspoon garlic powder or 2–5 garlic cloves, crushed
1/2–1 teaspoon cayenne (optional)

If you use fresh garlic, use up the dressing within two or three days. If you use garlic powder, the dressing will keep for a few weeks in the fridge.

Add three or four tablespoons of the dressing to each six cups (1.5 L) of salad.

Onion

1 chopped onion
1 chopped boiled egg
4 tablespoons olive oil
2 tablespoons apple cider vinegar
salt, pepper, dill, parsley

Lemony

2 tablespoons lemon juice
2 tablespoons olive oil
salt, pepper
1–2 garlic cloves, crushed

Lemony 2

juice of 2 lemons
1/4 teaspoons sugar
4–6 tablespoons olive oil

Dandelion coffee

Scrub autumn-dug roots with a brush (leave the root bark), remove any bad parts, and chop them into quarter-inch (1 cm) pieces. Let them dry until they're still a little moist, and then roast them in a dry cast iron pan, stirring often. Don't let the pieces get too dark, or they'll be very bitter. When they're evenly brown, they're done.

Grind roasted pieces in a coffee grinder and use as you would coffee. (For bonus points, find a cast-iron root-roaster and manual coffee grinder in Great-grandma's attic, and use those!)

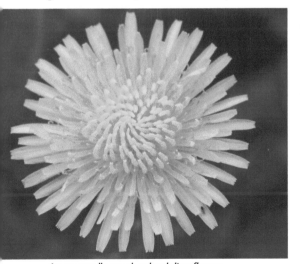

An unusually regular dandelion flower.

Boiled dandelion leaves

Bring dandelion leaf to a boil in water to cover, simmer for 10 minutes, and pour off the liquid. Repeat. If the taste is still too strong, repeat again. Cool and add some sour cream, a pinch of salt, and some lemon juice. Serve with croutons.

OTHER USES

Short-lived tattoos

You can use the white "milk" of the leaf, flower stalk, and root to make temporary tattoos. Try it on the inside of your arm. Your artwork won't be visible right away, though. Stay out of the shower, and by the next morning your now-brown "tattoo" will be there for all to see! The tattoo will last a few days, but you can wash it off whenever you like.

The bright yellow tattoos made from the juice of greater celandine (*Chelidonium majus*) will be visible immediately, but they won't last overnight.

The bright-orange juice of fresh California poppy root (*Eschscholzia californica*) works for tattoos, too, but it's even more short-lived than greater celandine's.

Although the juice of these plants has been used to eliminate warts, their tattoos are not irritating to the skin.

Wart removal

Apply the juice of any of the aforementioned tattoo plants to your wart a few times a day for a week or two.

The presence of many warts indicates that your immune system is having difficulty coping with viruses. Take St. John's wort internally, along with other immune-supporting herbs.

Some homeopaths believe that a single wart tells of a deeper imbalance, and if you remove the wart the imbalance will show in a less benign way.

Blow a fluffball

If you can blow all seeds from a dandelion puff in one breath, you may wish for something. (And you have very strong lungs.)

To better your chances, blow the fluff from the stem side. And choose a dry, almost overripe puff. If you still can't get all seeds to fly away, pick another and try again.

You'll improve your chances of getting your wish if you blow the seeds over an utterly dandelion-free lawn.

WARNINGS

Don't use dandelion or chicory regularly if you have low blood pressure, and avoid herbal coffees that include these herbs.

Both dandelion and chicory are strongly diuretic, which leads to lower blood pressure. You'll feel faint, you'll wilt in hot weather, you won't tolerate hot baths or saunas, and you can even start to keel over unless you stop using these herbs.

People with low blood pressure benefit from eating salt, vegetables, and proteins. They should exercise regularly and avoid sugar and other simple carbohydrates. And they should use fewer diuretic liver herbs.

As a bitter, dandelion increases bile secretion. It's not suited to people who have largish gall stones, though, as the bile can dislodge the stones.

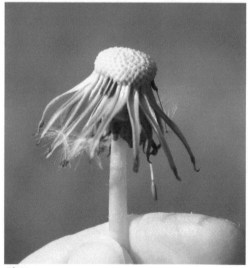

Blown.

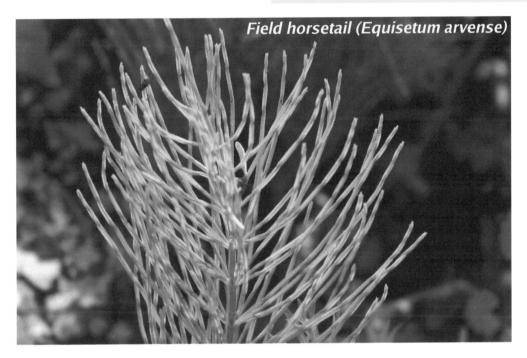

Field horsetail (Equisetum arvense)

FIELD HORSETAIL

An herb from the time of the dinosaurs.

***Equisetum arvense*:** Also called common horsetail, shave grass.

- Field horsetail (*Equisetum arvense*): Branches don't divide (much), and they usually point upward. The sheath on the main stem is shorter than the first joint of the side branches. The size of the branch sheaths is irrelevant. Field horsetail has two distinct shoots—the fertile brownish spring shoot and the sterile green summer shoot.

- Marsh horsetail (*Equisetum palustre*): Its main stem sheath is longer than the first joint of the branches. The size of the branch sheaths is irrelevant. The shoot bears a a cone-like structure at its tip, called a strobilus, in spring. This shrivels away once the green branches appear on the same shoot.

- Wood horsetail (*Equisetum sylvaticum*): The branches themselves branch profusely, usually pointing downward.

- Meadow horsetail (*Equisetum pratense*): The branches divide somewhat and are elegant and wavy.

- Water horsetail (*Equisetum fluviatile*): This horsetail grows in water and is rather large. Its main stem has few branches, and those it has are very short.

Family: Horsetail family, *Equisetaceae*

Perennial: Harvest in summer.

Cultivation: Gardeners curse this tenacious weed. Horsetail propagates via spores and thrives in acid soil. To get rid of it, you'll have to change the soil.

On the other hand, horsetail roots are so deep they bring up nutrients for other plants. Don't get rid of all your horsetail patches.

Tomato growers often are glad to have it. Horsetail contains a lot of potassium and makes an excellent garden cover.

Because horsetail is high in silica, it helps other plants repel fungal diseases.

Habitat: Horsetail is fond of ditches, fields, and moist meadows.

Appearance: The yellowish-brown spring shoot bears a strobilus or spore head at its tip. The green summer shoot is sterile; it resembles a small spruce, except its branches aren't divided.

Look-alikes: Other horsetail species. Mare's tail *(Hippuris* species) somewhat resembles this plant and is sometimes also called horsetail.

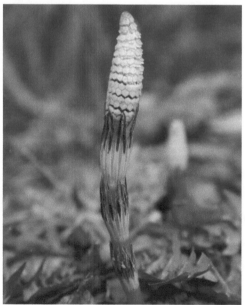

*The spring shoot of field horsetail (*Equisetum arvense).

78

In Finland, only field horsetail is considered nontoxic. In the U.S., any horsetail may be used.

Important constituents: Silica (7–10 %), potassium, other minerals and trace elements, flavonoids, saponins.

PICKING AND PROCESSING

The green shoots are best gathered in early to midsummer. The later you pick, the harder the horsetail gets, and the more difficult it becomes to get minerals out of it.

You can pick green shoots in September, but you'll need to boil them.

Remove dark brown and black parts and dry the shoots at room temperature out of the light.

Use them in teas, or make a vinegar from them.

EFFECTS AND USES

Horsetail is ideal for nail and hair problems.

(Brittle nails? Check your diet and digestion: why aren't food minerals being absorbed? Supplement with magnesium, potassium, calcium, zinc, vitamin B, C, D, and fish oils.

Fragile hair is often due to coloring chemicals. Refrain from coloring for a while, or switch to gentler hair products. Otherwise—again, check diet and digestion.)

Because horsetail contains silica, it speeds healing of broken bones.

The tincture of the green shoots is as effective for broken bones as the tea.

Horsetail is diuretic and styptic. It can be of help in respiratory and joint problems, and it strengthens connective tissue.

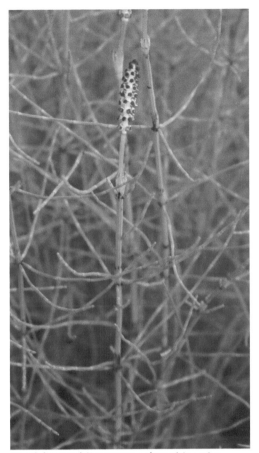

*Marsh horsetail (*Equisetum palustre*) in spring.*

A mineral-rich horsetail tea is useful during recuperation from illness or injury.

For joint pain, enjoy a hot horsetail bath, or make a hot compress.

Horsetail tea

1–2 teaspoons dried horsetail
  (picked fairly young)
1 cup (250 ml) boiling water

Pour water over the herb, steep for 15 minutes, and strain. Drink two to three cups a day.

Horsetail decoction

1–2 teaspoons dried horsetail
  (picked later in the season)
1 cup (250 ml) cold water

Add herb and water to a saucepan, bring to a boil, simmer for 15 minutes, and strain. Drink one or two cups a day for the minerals of horsetail.

Horsetail maceration

1–2 teaspoons dried herb
1 cup (250 ml) cold water
1/2 cup (125 ml) boiling water

Steep herb in the cold water for 10 to 15 hours. Add the boiling water and steep for 45 minutes more; strain. Drink two to three cups a day for joint problems, swellings, and long-term cough.

A tea blend for broken bones

1 teaspoon calendula or *Plantago* plantain
  leaf (they help heal)
1 teaspoon nettles, red raspberry leaf,
  or lady's mantle (they contain minerals)
1 teaspoon horsetail or green oats (they
  contain silica)
1 teaspoon meadowsweet (helps with pain)

Mix. Use 1–2 teaspoons of the mix to 1 cup (250 ml) boiling water, steep for 10 to 15 minutes, and strain. Drink up to three cups a day.

Horsetail tincture

4 ounces (100 g) fresh green shoots cut
  in 1/3–1-inch (1–3 cm) lengths
8 fluid ounces (200 ml) 190 proof grain
  alcohol (95 %)

Put the cut-up herb in a glass jar, cover with alcohol, and close the lid tightly. Steep two to four weeks. Strain, bottle, and label (example: "Horsetail, 1:2 95 %, 6.2021, my yard"). Dosage is 10–30 drops, up to three times a day.

Horsetail compress

handful dried horsetail
1 quart (liter) boiling water

Pour boiling water over the herb, steep until the liquid is just cool enough to be comfortable to the skin, and strain. Dip a towel or rag in the tea, and squeeze out excess liquid. Put the moist hot towel on the painful area, and leave it there for 30 to 40 minutes.

A horsetail bath

2 quarts (2 liters) boiling water
dried or fresh horsetail

Fresh herb: Cover herb with water.

Dried herb: Put herb in a pan and add triple the amount of water.

Bring to a boil, turn off heat, and steep for 20 to 30 minutes. Strain. Pour into bathwater and add enough cold water to make for a comfortable bath. Get in and enjoy!

OTHER USES

Dried horsetails have been used to polish metal vessels. Tin vessels in particular have received a scratchless shine with the help of horsetails.

Horsetail is excellent in footbaths.

Horsetail toothpowder

dried powdered horsetail

Use a pinch of the powder on a moistened toothbrush instead of toothpaste.

WARNINGS

Don't use horsetail as a diuretic if you have kidney- or bladderstones.

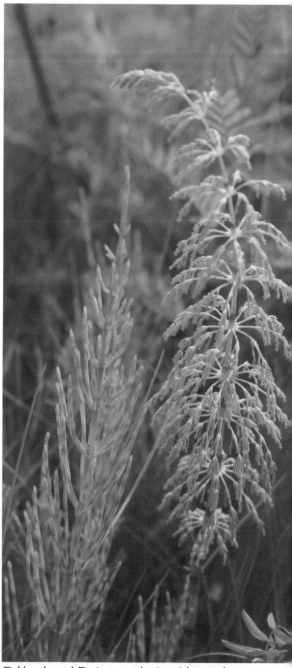

Field and wood (Equisetum sylvaticum) *horsetails.*

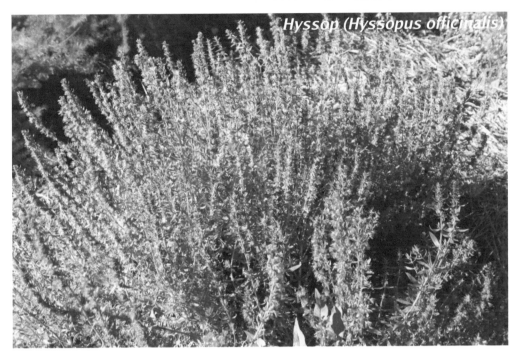
Hyssop (Hyssopus officinalis)

HYSSOP

If you want to be posh like they were in the 18th century, spread some hyssop on the floor. It releases a lovely scent when you tread on it, and no one will notice your dust bunnies.

Hyssopus officinalis

Family: Mint family, *Lamiaceae*

Perennial: Harvest from summer to fall.

Cultivation: You can grow hyssop from seeds or from cuttings. Hyssop is a short-lived perennial in the garden, but it self-seeds abundantly. Don't pull up all small seedlings—one sunny day you'll notice that your mother plant has died.

Hares take care of winter cuttings, at least up here. If they don't where you are, cut the plant to the ground in spring before it leafs out, or you'll end up with an unruly bush instead of the rounded garden beauty you're used to.

Grow hyssop in well-drained soil and give it some lime. Planted alone it makes a nice, hemispherical bush. In rows, it forms dense low hedges.

Appearance: Hyssop comes with blue, pink, or white flowers. Blue-flowering hyssop thrives in colder climates. Stems can grow to 18 inches (50 cm).

Notice the constant buzz around the flowering plants: honeybees, bumble-bees, and other pollinators love hyssop.

Important constituents: Essential oils, flavonoids, bitters, organic acids, tannins (5–8 %)

81

PICKING AND PROCESSING

Cut the flowering stems above the woody part. Bind into bundles of 8–15 stems and hang to dry in a shady spot.

Hyssop gathered after it has flowered won't be as strong, and the dried herb won't be as pretty.

Either cut the dried herb into 1-inch (2–3 cm) pieces (you'll need strong fingers), or strip the leaves and flowers from the stems (wear gloves). Store in airtight glass jars.

You also may use 2–4 inches (5–10 cm) of the fresh flowering tops.

EFFECTS AND USES

Hyssop is an aromatic, warming, anti-inflammatory, mint-family plant. Its essential oils help relieve menstrual and digestive cramps, its bitters help the digestion, and its tannins make it astringent.

Because it strengthens capillaries and increases peripheral blood supply, hyssop helps inflamed tissues heal faster.

Hyssop has been found to slow viral replication, especially in the lungs. It helps you sweat and is diuretic. (If you tend to sweat a lot anyway, however, it won't make you sweat even more.)

A hot tea of hyssop is good for coughs, flu, digestive problems such as irritable bowel, and urinary tract infections. Gargled, it's one of our best remedies for a sore throat.

Hyssop is a pleasant tea for those recuperating from flu.

Hyssop salve applied to chest and back soothes coughs. Use it for bruises,

sprains, muscle pain, and insect bites, as well. Out of salve? A fresh-hyssop compress—or just the fresh crushed leaves—will treat muscle pain, bruises, and swellings.

And try a hyssop bath—especially for joint pain!

Hyssop tea

1–2 teaspoons dried hyssop
1 cup (250 ml) boiling water

Pour boiling water over the herb, steep for 10 minutes, strain.

The flavor is a little lemony and aromatic. Drink two to three cups a day.

Hyssop compress

1 handful dried hyssop
or 2 handfuls fresh
1 quart (liter) boiling water

Pour the water over the herb, steep 15 minutes, strain, and cool just until it can be comfortably applied to skin. Dip a cloth or small towel in the tea, and squeeze out excess liquid. Put the moist, hot towel on the painful area and leave it there for 30 to 40 minutes.

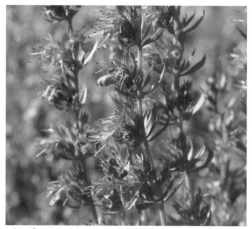

Blue-flowering hyssop.

Oil and salve of hyssop

Make an herbal oil from the dried herb (page 18), and use it to make a salve (page 22).

Apply to the back and chest for coughs, or apply to bruises, sprains, muscle aches, and insect bites.

A hyssop bath

2 quarts (2 liters) water
dried or fresh hyssop

Cover the fresh herb with water. (If you use dried herb, use three times as much water.)

Bring to a boil, steep for 15 minutes, strain, and pour into bathwater. Add enough cold water to make for a comfortable bath. Get in the tub and enjoy!

FOOD USES

Add hyssop (especially the fresh tops) to stews, meat, pasta, soups, sauces, and salads.

The flowering tops are nice in fruit salads.

Hyssop makes a tasty tea. The dried herb's hint of lemon makes it even better.

An herbal spread

3–4 tablespoons fresh minced herbs
(hyssop, caraway leaf, tarragon, thyme, lovage, parsley and/or dill)
1/4 teaspoon salt
1 cup (250 ml) sour cream or Greek yogurt

Mix. Serve on bread. Yum!

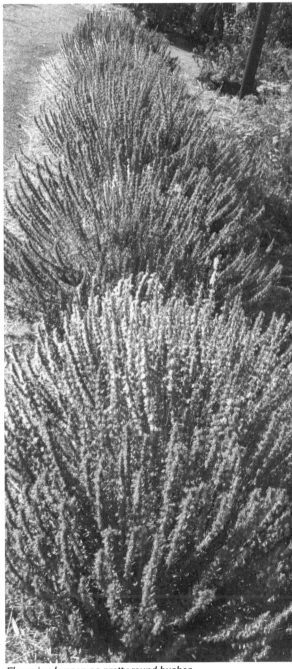

Flowering hyssop as pretty round bushes.

83

MINT-FAMILY ANTI-INFLAMMATORY PLANTS

Herb books often refer to this or that plant as "anti-inflammatory." And more often than not, this plant will be in the mint family (*Lamiaceae*).

So if a formula calls for, say, oregano (*Origanum* species), and you have none on hand, you can safely replace it with herbs such as ground ivy (*Glechoma hederacea*), hemp nettle (*Galeopsis* species), rosemary (*Rosmarinus officinalis*), the spicy sages (*Salvia* species), marjoram (*Origanum majorana*), bee balm (*Monarda* species), or basil (*Ocimum* species).

If you're advised to take a woundwort or hedgenettle (*Stachys* or *Betonica* species), and, because you don't know the plant, you haven't any, you may replace it with herbs such as all-heal (*Prunella vulgaris*), hyssop (*Hyssopus officinalis*), giant hyssop (*Agastache* species), thyme (*Thymus* species)—or oregano, ground ivy, hemp nettle, and the like.

Note the nuances in anti-inflammatory qualities of these herbs.

For example, ground ivy (*Glechoma hederacea*) is first-rate for inflammations of facial mucous membranes.

Hyssop is very good for throat irritation.

Sage, the monardas, and thyme shine for lung problems.

The culinary herbs basil, rosemary, oregano, and marjoram are also useful for intestinal troubles.

Nuances aside, though, just remember that in a pinch you can replace any of these with any other.

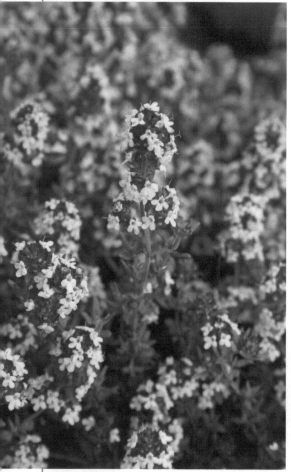

Thyme in full flower.

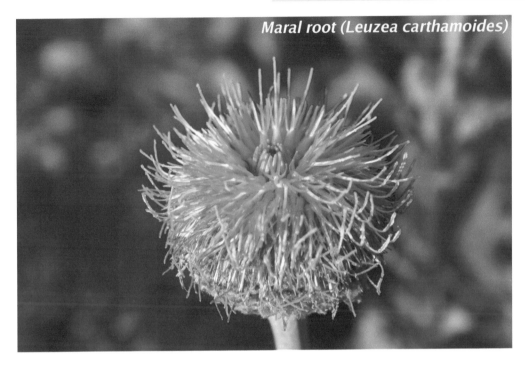

Maral root (Leuzea carthamoides)

MARAL ROOT

Great for strengthening the kidneys and the adrenals, and beautiful too.

Leuzea carthamoides (*Rhaponticum carthamoides, Stemmacantha carthamoides*): Also called Russian leuzea

Family: Daisy family, *Asteraceae*

Perennial: Harvest in fall.

Habitat: Native to the subalpine zone (4,500–6,000 feet above sea level) and alpine meadows of Siberia and Kazakhstan, maral root must be grown in cultivation elsewhere.

Cultivation: Maral root seeds require the cold of winter to germinate. They remain viable for years. Sow in fall or spring in sandy or similarly loose soil. Avoid planting in clay soils if you aim to harvest roots.

Appearance: The leaves are grayish green, deeply divided, on stems that can grow as tall as 36 inches (1 meter). The flower stalk rises to a height of about 5 feet (1.5 m). Maral root flowers at the beginning of June. The flowers are an inch and a half across (5 cm) by an inch and a third (4 cm) in length. The roots are slender, very tough, and colored dark brown or black. They're attached to a central piece that's around a half-inch (1–2 cm) in diameter.

Look-alikes: Maral root blossoms somewhat resemble thistle blossoms.

Important constituents: Ecdysteroids (0.1–0.7% in the root, 0.01–0.1% in the leaf, 2% in the seed); flavonoids, glycosides, and sesquiterpene lactones in the root

PICKING AND PROCESSING

It's easy to dig the roots in sandy soil. I haven't heard of anyone who's managed to get them out of clay.

The Russian literature recommends digging the roots at the end of the second year. I dig mine when they're about three years old.

Use an axe or billhook machete to chop the root ball to pieces. Rinse off the larger debris, pull the roots into smaller pieces, and remove any remaining small stones, earthworms, and foreign root matter. Cut the thicker roots into quarter-inch (5 mm) pieces. Dry below 104 °F (40 °C) and store in airtight jars.

EFFECTS AND USES

This plant is a real adaptogen. It enhances one's overall performance, general well-being, immune system, and stress tolerance. It also strengthens nerves and helps you think better.

Maral root is excellent if you have low blood pressure with pale urine. Because strengthened kidneys make less urine, your low blood pressure will rise—important if you can't take heat. If all the liquids you drink end up in your pee, you have nothing left to sweat with. Your heat regulation on warm days (or in the sauna) just isn't there, and you suffer. You can feel faint, dizzy, or light-headed.

Maral root helps with low blood pressure for as long as you keep taking it.

People with low blood pressure also should exercise, eat more greens, proteins, and fat, and salt their food.

The root improves sleep quality dramatically in overly stressed people. A good night's sleep ensures quality work the next day, and stress is reduced by that much.

Maral root strengthens adrenals and helps with exhaustion. But don't depend on it alone to get you through. If you're on the verge of burnout, you also should stop taking stimulants such as coffee, guarana, cola nuts, and energy drinks. Real burnout can take years to come back from. Remember—graveyards are full of indispensable people.

Maral root helps treat impotence, but note that the best cure for impotence is a good workout a few times a week: it'll stiffen and get to orgasm.

This herb speeds wound healing and recovery from illness and childbirth. It also protects against some side effects of steroid medication.

A decoction of maral root is helpful in treating alcoholism. Take half a glassful four to five times a day for several months. (It helps to attend AA meetings and follow other recommended protocols.)

You can use the root in teas or tinctures. Tea can be made from the leaf, but it's much weaker in effect. I've given the seeds, as well, as a tea or to chew on.

Tea of maral root leaf

1–2 teaspoons dried leaves
1 cup (250 ml) boiling water

Pour boiling water over the herb, steep for 10 minutes, and strain. Drink up to three cups a day.

Maral root decoction

1–2 teaspoons dried roots in small pieces
1 cup (250 ml) cold water

Put herb and water in a pan, bring to a boil, simmer for 10 minutes, and strain. Drink up to three cups a day.

Maral root tincture

From fresh root:

4 ounces (100 g) fresh roots in 1/3–1-inch (1–3 cm) pieces
8 fluid ounces (200 ml) 190 proof grain alcohol (95 %)

From dried root:

4 ounces (100 g) fresh roots in 1/3–1-inch (1–3 cm) pieces
20 fluid ounces (500 ml) 100 proof grain alcohol (50 %)

Put the root bits in a glass jar, cover with the alcohol, and close the lid tightly. Steep for two to four weeks, strain, bottle, and label (example: "Maral root, 1:5 50 %, 04.2021, purchased").

Dosage is 30–60 drops, up to three times daily.

To help with childbirth, take 30–60 drops an hour for three hours.

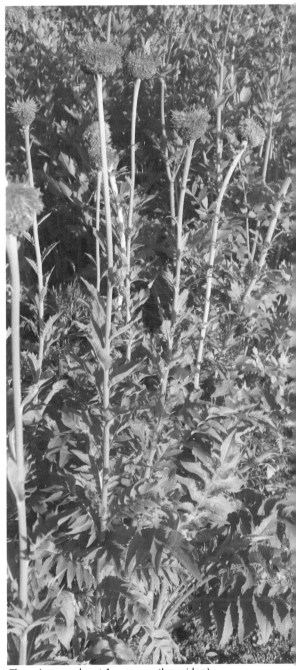

Flowering maral root (Leuzea carthamoides).

DIGESTIVE UPSET

Inappropriate food can give you a stomachache. Rancid fat makes for a really uncomfortable feeling. The cramping before a major gas eruption is painful, as well.

So it's a good thing, then, that help is as near as your own spice shelf—because of course you have caraway!

Just chew 5–10 caraway seeds to calm your stomach and end the griping. That uncomfortable feeling will stop, too, and the gas eruption will be rather milder.

No caraway? Try aniseed, fennel seed, or coriander or dill seed. Or, if you know your umbellifers, grab a few seeds of a wild angelica or other edible carrot-family plant.

They all work for this kind of short-lived gut upset.

It's possible to prevent gas, too. In Germany, cabbage- and onion-based recipes often call for caraway seeds to prevent flatulence.

Persistent digestive upset calls for a visit to the doctor.

NAUSEA

Ginger in any form will relieve nausea, whether chewed raw or taken as tea, ginger ale, ginger snaps, or ginger candy. They all work pretty fast.

Ginger helps with motion sickness in both children and adults, and it works for the nausea of pregnancy and after you've feasted a little too well at holiday time.

If you have no ginger, try thyme instead—chew a few leaves, or make a thyme tea. It won't be as effective as ginger, but it will provide some relief.

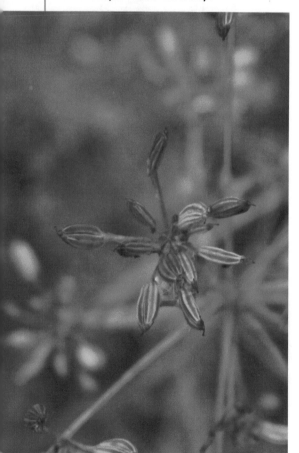

Caraway seeds.

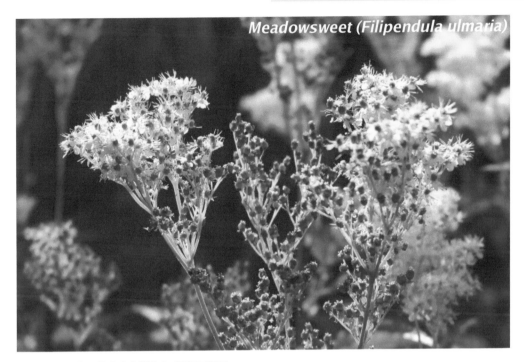
Meadowsweet (Filipendula ulmaria)

MEADOWSWEET

A splendid pain reliever.

Filipendula ulmaria: Also called queen of the meadow and brideswort

Family: Rose family, *Rosaceae*

Perennial: Harvest in summer.

Habitat: Meadowsweet thrives in damp meadows and drainage ditches and alongside rivers and lakes.

Appearance: The creamy white, somewhat irregular flowerheads are quite showy in July.

Look-alikes: Other species of *Filipendula*; the unscented ones, such as dropwort (*Filipendula vulgaris*), can't be used like meadowsweet. Use the scented ones instead.

Important constituents: Salicylates, flavonoids, vitamins; up to 10 % tannins (green parts); also mucilage, sugars (flower buds and flowers)

PICKING AND PROCESSING

Pick the flowering tops of meadowsweet by breaking off their stalks beneath the lowermost blossoms.

Leave any plants that are covered in powdery mildew; meadowsweets in drier and less densely populated spots are less likely to have fungal diseases.

To dry, spread your harvest on clean old cotton sheets over a layer of news-papers, hang bundles indoors out of the light, or use a dehydrator set below 104 °F (40 °C).

The plant's flower bud is the strongest part, after that the flowers, and finally the green parts.

You may encounter a color-changing spider on some meadowsweet flowers. Leave them: the spider was there first.

Any meadowsweet part is suitable for external uses (footbath, infused oil, salve, and so on).

To prepare the herb for internal applications, use the flowers and flower buds. They contain mucilage and sugars that soften the plant's otherwise harsh acids and tannins. Greens will only irritate mucous membranes.

The root of meadowsweet is a 2.5- to 3-inch (6–7 cm) tube with walls only 1 mm or so in thickness. From it spring a handful of rootlets barely a tenth of an inch (2–3 mm) across and about 2 inches (5 cm) long (you wonder how the plant manages to stay upright!).

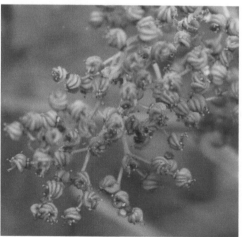

*The interesting seeds of meadowsweet (*Filipendula ulmaria*).*

But don't bother digging the roots. It's a lot of work for yet another harsh salicylate plant part.

EFFECTS AND USES

Meadowsweet in baths, footbaths, compresses, oils, and salves is excellent for treating a variety of aches and pains.

It's useful for pain taken internally, too, but remember: pain is the body telling you to slow down.

Although you can use meadowsweet to treat transient headaches, it's better to find a chronic headache's cause and remedy that. Are your neck muscles too tight? Are you tired? Dehydrated? Do you have sinusitis? Are your glasses right for your eyes? Do you have a fever? Did you skip your usual cuppa coffee? Is your blood sugar low? Did you drink too much last night? Is it migraine, a brain tumor, or something else?

Meadowsweet is commonly used for the aches and pains of a real flu, but consider the following.

First, using nonsteroidal anti-inflammatory drugs, or NSAIDs (including meadowsweet), hampers your immune system.

Second, relieving flu discomfort means you'll have to keep reminding yourself to stay in bed.

Third, if you disregard the aches and get up too soon after a good bout of flu, you risk getting bronchitis—or, worse, pneumonia. (People don't usually die of the flu itself; they die of just such complications.)

Finally, if you engage in vigorous activity too soon after a flu you can get myocarditis, which can be really nasty.

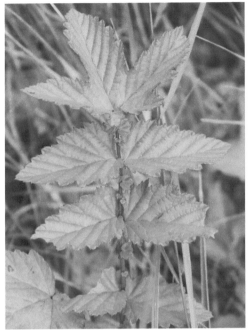

A leaf of meadowsweet. Notice the tiny leaflets that sprout between the larger ones, and the stem's three-leafed tip.

I like meadowsweet for respiratory ailments primarily because it can bring on a sweat, and that can lower a too-high fever. Yarrow is another effective sweat-inducer. A combination of these two works very well.

A tea of meadowsweet flowers or flower buds is good for stomach and duodenal ulcers: they contain mucilage (which protects the stomach lining), their tannins help shrink mildly congested tissue, and their salicylates are anti-inflammatory.

These days science blames the bacterium *Helicobacter pylori* for most stomach ulcers, but a stressful lifestyle or overuse of NSAIDs (aspirin, ibuprofen, and the like) can render the body vulnerable in the first place.

Duodenal ulcers can result from acid-producing stomach cells sitting on the wrong side of the sphincter.

Other herbs for ulcers include calendula and *Plantago* species (which help heal damaged tissues); mallow leaf, root, and flower (which contribute protective mucilage), and the leaf of red raspberry or rosebay willowherb (which is mildly astringent).

A bath of meadowsweet relaxes the muscles and relieves pain.

Meadowsweet tea

1 teaspoon dried or fresh meadowsweet flowers or flower buds
1 cup (250 ml) boiling water

Pour boiling water over the herb, steep for 5 minutes, and strain. Drink up to three cups a day, as needed.

Meadowsweet tea tastes good, unless you once make it too strong and drink it anyway. After that, its scent and taste will repel you for years.

Meadowsweet compress

1 handful dried meadowsweet
or 2 handfuls fresh
1 quart (liter) boiling water

Pour the boiling water over the herb, steep for 15 minutes, strain, and let cool until just skin-comfortable. Dip a towel or rag in the tea, and squeeze out excess liquid. Put the moist, hot towel on the achy spot, and leave it for 30 to 40 minutes.

Oil and salve of meadowsweet

Make an herbal oil from the dried herb (page 18), and then make a salve from the oil (page 22).

Apply to achy or painful areas.

91

A meadowsweet footbath

dried or fresh meadowsweet

Fresh: Put the herb in a 1-quart (liter) pan and add water to cover.

Dried: Put the herb in a 1-quart (liter) pan and add three times as much water.

Bring to a boil, steep for 15 minutes, and strain. Pour into a basin or large bowl and add cold water to cool to a comfortable temperature. Put your feet in for 10 to 20 minutes. Remember to wriggle your toes in delight from time to time!

A meadowsweet bath

dried or fresh meadowsweet

Fresh: Put the herb in a 2-quart (2-liter) pan and add water to cover.

Dried: Put the herb in a 2-quart (2-liter) pan and add triple the amount of water.

Bring to a boil, steep for 15 minutes, strain, and add to bathwater. Adjust the temperature for comfort, get in, and enjoy!

USES IN MAINSTREAM MEDICINE

Aspirin got its name from meadowsweet: the 'a' comes from acetyl salicylic acid, the "spirin" comes from the old name for meadowsweet, *Spiraea ulmaria*. (Salicylic acid, of course, got its name from the Latin name for willows, Salix.)

FOOD USES

Rub the interior of your brewing vessel with fresh meadowsweet flowers to add spice to beer, wine, and mead.

WARNINGS

Some asthmatics and anyone sensitive to aspirin must avoid meadowsweet and other plants high in salicylates.

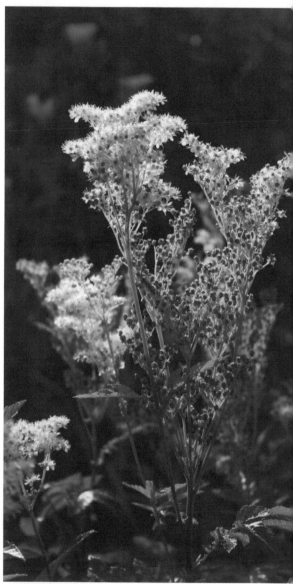

Meadowsweet flower.

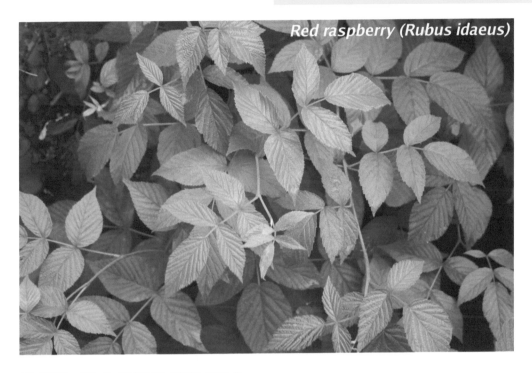

Red raspberry (Rubus idaeus)

RED RASPBERRY

An herb for pregnancy and menstrual problems.

***Rubus idaeus*:** Also called raspberry, European red raspberry

Family: Rose family, *Rosaceae*

Perennial: Biennial stalks. Harvest in spring to early summer (leaves), summer (berries).

Habitat: Red raspberry is among the first plants to recolonize cut or burned forests.

Cultivation: Red raspberry generally will flower and fruit on last year's stalks, so if you want berries, don't cut down the whole plant in late fall or early spring.

Some cultivars will flower and fruit on this year's stalks, though.

You'll get more raspberries if you grow yellow-berried cultivars; the birds aren't as interested in them. Some cultivars require a winter net to deter hungry hares.

Appearance: The stalks are straight, unbranched, and with large leaves in the first year. During the second year the stalks branch and flower; they have more spines, and the leaves are smaller. The underside of the leaf is pale to nearly white.

Look-alikes: Other species of *Rubus*. Their berries are edible and the leaf can often (but not always) be used as herbal teas.

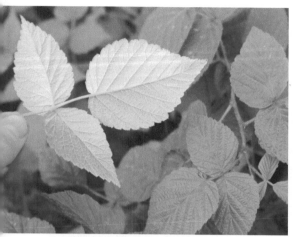
A red raspberry leaf from beneath.

Important constituents: Tannins, flavonoids, plant acids, vitamin C (leaves); fruit acids (including citric acid), sugars, flavonoids, pectin, essential oil (fruit)

PICKING AND PROCESSING

Harvest the leaves or the whole first-year stalks around midsummer, when they're fully grown but still healthy and clean. Spread the leaves on a cotton sheet or in a dehydrator set to 85–105° F (30–40° C). Bundle the stalks and hang them to dry out of the light in a well-ventilated room.

You may use the leaves of cultivars, provided they're grown organically.

EFFECTS AND USES

Because red raspberry belongs to the rose family, its leaves belong to the rose-family astringents (page 96). That's why a tea of the leaves has been useful to remedy diarrhea, inflamed gums, and eczema, among other things. The tea, gargled, also helps with throat problems.

The leaves are rich in minerals and trace elements.

The tea is excellent for ladies. It fortifies the pelvic organs, which makes it helpful for a variety of menstrual problems—too much, too little, too seldom, too frequent, too painful, and so on.

Raspberry leaf tea is also effective for many cervical issues. If a pap smear indicates trouble, drink raspberry leaf tea for a few weeks. Often a subsequent test will be clean. (A simple vitamin B deficiency, especially B6, can cause pap smear abnormalities. Take your Bs—and some magnesium to help absorption—and reduce your intake of sweets, sodas, fruit juices, and similar sugary treats.)

Red raspberry leaf provides support during pregnancy, both because of its mineral content, and because it strengthens the pelvic organs. However, it may cause spotting during the first three months; although this isn't dangerous, it can be worrisome, so wait until your second trimester to start drinking the tea.

And keep drinking red raspberry leaf tea after giving birth. It speeds recuperation.

A tea or vinegar made from the berries is helpful in lowering a too-high fever.

Red raspberry leaf tea

1 teaspoon dried red raspberry leaves
or 2 teaspoons fresh leaves
1 cup (250 ml) boiling water

Pour boiling water over the herb and steep for 10 minutes. Strain through a coffee filter. Drink two or three cups a day for many weeks.

Switch to lady's mantle if you grow tired of the taste of red raspberry.

Red raspberry leaf decoction

5 teaspoons dried leaves
1 cup (250 ml) cold water

Add herb and water to a pan, bring to a boil, simmer for 10 minutes, and strain through a coffee filter. Drink one to three cups a day in small sips for diarrhea or similar gut problems.

Wash your mouth with the cooled tea two to four times a day until sore mucous membranes have healed, or use it externally for skin rashes and eczema.

Red raspberry tea

2–4 teaspoons fresh berries
1 cup (250 ml) boiling water

Pour water over the herb, steep for 10 minutes, and strain. Let cool somewhat, and drink two or three cups a day for fever.

Raspberry vinegar

4 ounces (100 g) fresh berries
1 cup (250 ml) apple cider vinegar

Pour the berries into a glass jar and add vinegar to cover. Cover the jar's mouth with plastic wrap, and then with a lid. (A metal lid will corrode in contact with vinegar.) Steep in a dark spot for two weeks. Strain, bottle, and label (example: "Raspberry vinegar, July 2021").

A tablespoon of the red raspberry vinegar drunk in a glass of water helps reduce the heat of excessive sweating and fever.

Use small amounts in salads or bouillons.

If you store the vinegar in a dark, cool place, it will retain its color and flavor for about a year.

FOOD USES

You can use the leaves of spineless red raspberry cultivars as you would spinach.

The leaves—fresh or dried, as-is or fermented (see page 14)—make a pleasant herbal tea.

Raspberry leaf spinach

Rinse and chop the fresh (spineless) leaves. Add butter to a pan and fry some onions until soft. Add the chopped leaves, and let them soften a bit. Add flour and cream to taste. Finish with some salt and nutmeg, and serve.

OTHER USES

Astringent herbs—red raspberry leaf among them—are useful as a facial wash. The scent is always a nice bonus.

WARNINGS

Always strain anything you make from red raspberry leaf through a coffee filter. The leaves' undersides are studded with tiny spines that can irritate mucous membranes.

Avoid consuming red raspberry leaf during the first trimester of pregnancy.

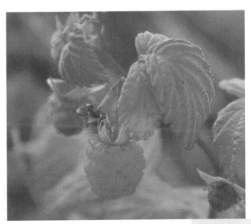

ROSE-FAMILY ASTRINGENT PLANTS

Almost every book on the uses of medicinal herbs offers up statements such as "Strawberry leaf helps with diarrhea," "Red raspberry leaf is great for inflamed gums," or "A tea of potentilla leaf works wonders for sunburned skin."

But these books often fail to point out the fact that all of these are mildly astringent rose-family herbs. And there are more.

Try, for instance, one or the other avens (*Geum* species), agrimony (*Agrimonia* species), lady's mantle (*Alchemilla*

*The flower of water or purple avens (*Geum rivale*).*

species), spirea (*Spiraea* species), rose (*Rosa* species), raspberries in general (*Rubus* species), and rowan or mountain ash (*Sorbus* species).

You'll find astringent herbs in other plant families, too. The geraniums (*Geranium* species), for example, are very effective, as is regular, store-bought black tea (*Camellia sinensis*) (although black tea isn't all that mild).

Astringent herbs pull together swelled mucosa or skin tissue. That's why they help with inflammation, and why they stop bacteria from wreaking havoc in those tissues.

Astringent herbs differ from anti-inflammatory herbs in that the astringents work only locally. They're useful both externally (on the skin) and internally (for problems in the whole length of the digestive tract).

Astringents won't help you with your cough or your UTIs, however; their tannins simply can't reach the inflamed tissues of lungs or bladder. They go from your mouth to your anus and can't deviate from that route.

Thus, if you read that strawberry leaf works for diarrhea, you may substitute any other astringent herb.

Rose-family astringents usually have a pleasant taste, and they can be found both in gardens and in the wild.

And if you can't find anything at all just now, use black tea, instead.

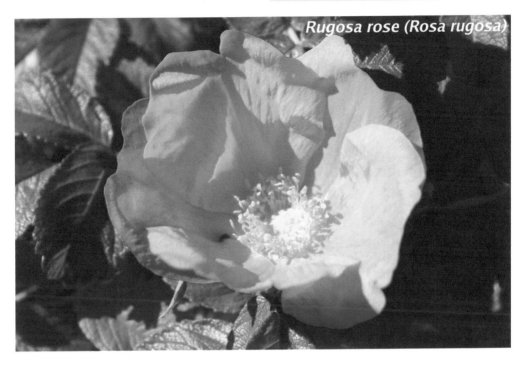

Rugosa rose (Rosa rugosa)

ROSE

A lovely, soothing, and mood-lifting flower.

Rosa species

Family: Rose family, *Rosaceae*

Perennial: Harvest in summer (petals) or fall (fruit).

Habitat: Wild roses thrive in a variety of environments. The cinnamon rose (*Rosa majalis*) is found along the edges of deciduous forests, in ditches, and next to cliffs. Rugosa rose (*Rosa rugosa*) runs wild along sandy coasts, ditches, and waysides.

Cultivation: Give fertilizer, sun, and porous soil to your roses.

Important constituents: Essential oils, flavonoids (flower petals); vitamins C, E, thiamine (B1), riboflavin (B2), and niacin (B3), fruit sugars, pectin, fruit acids, flavonoids, calcium (hips)

PICKING AND PROCESSING

The petals

Many of our pretty hybrid garden roses have no scent. They can't be used for our purposes.

Flower-shop roses are heavily sprayed; they can't be used, either.

Smell the roses in your garden: if the flowers have a heavenly scent, you can use them. Harvest the petals of strongly scented species in full flower.

97

If you're strongly allergic to insect stings, check each flower for pollinators before you pluck it.

Let them wilt for a day or two before you dry them to ensure a stronger scent in the dried petals.

Spread the petals on a cotton sheet to dry, or use a dehydrator set lower than 95 °F (35 °C). Store the dried petals in an airtight jar in a dark place.

Double-flowered scented species provide a lot of petals very quickly. Take only the petals, which are easily plucked. The remaining flower parts will become a rosehip, given the chance. Including the entire flower makes for slower drying, and they simply don't work as well as petals alone. They do have a strong apple scent, though, so you might dry some "flower bottoms" separately to make an apple-scented tea.

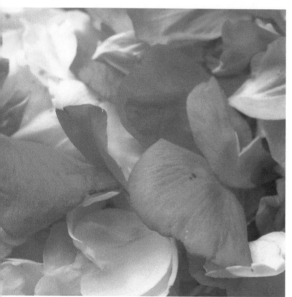

The rose species you use don't matter, as long as the petals are scented.

The hips

Pick the ripe rosehips (rose fruit) in autumn. Gather them before a hard frost, when they're still hard. Soft rosehips are hard to slice.

If you find a bush loaded with large rosehips, you'll fill your basket in no time. The largest rosehips come from Rugosa roses, but you can use any rose fruit you can find.

Cut into a handful or so of rosehips before you start really picking. This will give you an idea of the larvae population. If every hip has extra moving parts, move to the next bush (or the next rose species) and check that. Don't bother checking for bore holes; the flowery end of the hip is wide-open to insects.

To dry the hips in pieces, first remove the stalks and flower-side leaf rosettes. Then slice the hips into at least four parts. Dry in a dehydrator, or spread them to dry on a clean old bedsheet laid over a layer of newspapers.

To dry them whole, remove the stalk, but don't damage the hip. Leave the flowery leaf rosette; it hastens drying. Remove any dried petals that may still be attached.

Thread a needle with uncolored cotton thread and string the berries one by one, leaving a little space between them to prevent spoilage. Hang the laden threads to dry. If you have a lot of rosehip threads, this is very pretty. When your strung rosehips are very dry, remove any spoiled hips, and then slice each one open and discard any that have mold inside. Pour the good hips into your blender and give them a twirl.

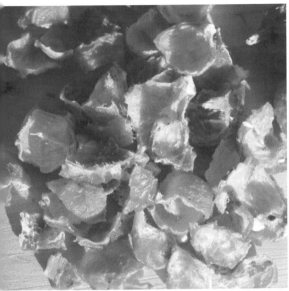

Sliced dried rosehips. There are some seeds—and some itchy hairs.

Getting rid of the itchy hairs

If you don't find the hairs itchy, you can leave the seeds with their hairs in the dried rosehips.

Removing hairs from fresh rosehips: Use a knife to dig out the seeds, including their hairs, from the hips. Wear protective gloves, or your nails will itch for a week afterward.
Remove the flower-side leaves, slice the berries, and boil them. Strain through cheesecloth.

Removing the hairs from dried rosehips: Shake the dried hip pieces outdoors, in a sieve, with the wind at your back (the seed hairs really do itch!).

EFFECTS AND USES
The petals

Rose petals are calming and mood-lifting. They help with anger and frustration, give you courage to defend your opinions and boundaries, and help you like yourself and others more. (But remember to let go of stress, and include some opportunities for rest and relaxation in your life.)

Rose can even help you reclaim your lost sexuality.

Use the petals in teas, tinctures, syrups, elixirs, baths, honeys, and so on.

Use rose petals for menstrual irritability. Drink a rose tea, take a rose bath—and take magnesium supplements and liver-strengthening herbs.

Drink rose tea for menstrual cramps, for mild gastric upset, and for coughs.

Try rose petals for irregular menses.

Garden sage tea helps with the hot flushes of menopause; add some rose to it, and you'll be able to relax about it all. Stressing out just worsens menopausal problems.

A paste of rose and honey soothes sore throats.

To treat diarrhea, drink a tea of rose buds or flowers every two or three hours.

Rose petals soothe the skin and help heal small wounds.

Let your rose petal tea go cold, and use it as a skin or face wash.

Rose vinegar calms sunburned skin, helps heal small wounds, and stops excessive sweating. Use it for basic skin care and for bruises, sprains, and the like.

The hips

Use rosehips if you're tired or exhausted, as a source of vitamin C, and when you must recuperate from an ordeal.

Rosehips can help with dry skin.

Externally, tea of rosehips used in a compress or as a wash can help heal wounds. (Remember to strain the tea through a coffee filter first, though, to get rid of the itchy hairs.)

Rose petal tea

1 teaspoon dried petals
or 2 teaspoons crushed fresh petals
1 cup (250 ml) boiling water

Pour boiling water over the herb, steep for 10 minutes, strain. Drink one to three cups a day.

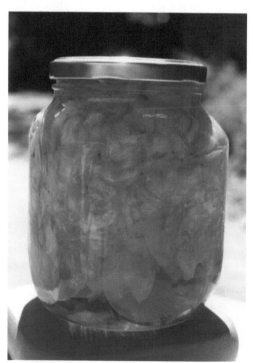

Rose petals steeping in vodka.

A tea of rose petals may taste of perfume, but it's an effective mood-lifter. It's also relaxing and helps with mild stomach and menstrual cramps.

Rose petal decoction

2–3 tablespoons fresh rose petals
1 cup (250 ml) cold water

Add the herb and water to a pan, bring to a boil, remove from heat, steep for 15 minutes, and strain.

Effective as a gargle for sore throat or inflamed mouth mucosa. Use as a wash for slow-healing sores and burns.

Rose petal elixir

That utterly undrinkable, high-alcohol clear liquid your Central European friends brought you years ago, with the weird fruit name you can't find in any dictionary? That's brandy, and that's excellent for elixirs.

fresh rose petals
liquid honey
brandy (or vodka)

Fill a glass jar with the petals. Add liquid honey to one-third of the jar. Then fill the jar with the brandy (or, in a pinch, vodka).

Steep for two to four weeks out of the light. Strain.

Take one or two teaspoons when the world is falling over you, when you want some smiles in your life, or when your nerves yearn for a holiday. Take a teaspoon when you need some courage or love, or you wish to show some thorns to the world.

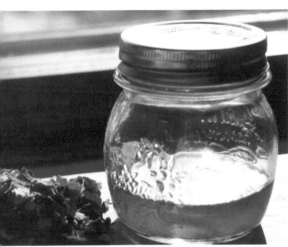

Rose petal vinegar from dried petals.

Rose vinegar

  dried rose petals
  apple cider vinegar or diluted white vinegar

Fill a glass jar one-quarter full of dried rose petals, and fill the rest with vinegar. Cover the mouth of the jar with plastic wrap, and carefully screw on the lid. (Vinegar will corrode a metal lid.) Leave in a dark spot for two weeks, strain, and bottle.

Use for small wounds and (especially) for itchy skin. Rose vinegar gives relief and a nice scent.

For use on young children, first dilute the vinegar 1:10–1:5.

Diluted 1:20, applications of rose vinegar help with excessive sweating.

Rose petal vodka

  fresh rose petals
  vodka (or brandy)

Fill a glass jar with fresh petals, cover with the alcohol, and close the lid. Steep two to four weeks, and strain. Use as you would rose elixir.

Rosebud tea

  5–10 rosebuds or whole rose flowers
  2 cups (500 ml) boiling water

Pour boiling water over the herb, steep for 20 minutes, and strain. Drink for diarrhea, or cool and use as a wash.

Rose-honey paste

From fresh petals:

  fresh rose petals
  liquid honey

Crush the petals into honey with a spoon to make a paste.

From dried petals:

  dried rose petals
  honey

Warm the honey in a waterbath until it's as runny as water. Add finely powdered dried petals to make a rather stiff paste. Take one or two tablespoons for a sore throat or to lift your mood.

Stored in an airtight jar, the paste will keep for years.

A rose petal bath

  2 quarts (2 liters) water
  dried or fresh rose petals

Fresh herb: Cover the herb with water.

Dried herb: Put the herb in a pan, and add three times as much water.

Bring to a boil, cover, and steep for 5 minutes. Strain and pour into bathwater. Add enough cold water to make a comfortable bath.

The only thing more luxurious than a rose-petal bath would be Cleopatra's legendary bath of donkey milk.

Rosehip decoction

2 teaspoons crushed dried rosehips
1 cup (250 ml) cold water

Add hips and water to a pan, bring to a boil, and simmer for 10 minutes. Strain through a coffee filter.

This decoction contains vitamin C, and it strengthens the immune system. Drink one to three cups a day, or more if you have the flu.

The vitamin C content stays high even after boiling. You can keep the tea with you in a Thermos bottle.

Storebought rosehip tea gets its color and taste from roselle (also called "jamaica" or "karkade"), which is the sour, deep red calyx of a *Hibiscus* species. You'd have to use large amounts of rosehips get the same flavor from your own rosehip tea.

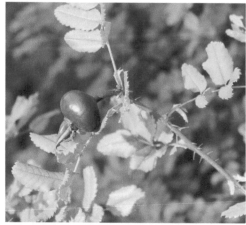

*The black rosehip of a burnet rose (*Rosa pimpinellifolia*).*

Rosehip puree

fresh rosehips

Remove stems and leaves, slice the hips in half, and scrape out the seeds and hairs (see page 99).

Rinse the hips a few times to dislodge the last few hairs. Pour them into a pan, add water to cover, and simmer them until they're soft.

Rub them through a sieve or food mill.

Freeze the puree in half-cup or 1-cup containers; 2 pounds (1 kg) rosehips makes about a quart (liter) of puree.

To sweeten your puree, add 2–8 ounces (50–200 grams) sugar or honey per quart (or liter) of puree, and simmer until the sugar has dissolved.

To spice it up, add a teaspoon cinnamon, 1–2 teaspoons ginger, or a pinch of nutmeg or allspice to each cup of puree.

Take a teaspoon of puree three to five times a day for the C vitamin, as a treat, as a nutritious strengthener, or to stimulate appetite.

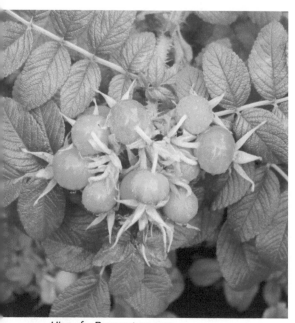

Hips of a Rugosa-type rose.

Rosehip compress

1 handful dried rosehips
or 2 handfuls fresh
1 quart (liter) boiling water

Pour boiling water over the herb, steep for 15 minutes, strain through a coffee filter, and cool until just skin-comfortable. Dip a towel or rag in the tea, and squeeze out excess liquid. Put the moist, hot towel on the painful area, and leave it there 30–40 minutes.

FOOD USES

You can eat rosehips straight off the bush, but nibble only the flesh. Your mouth may not itch after eating whole rosehips, but the other end might later on.

Use dried rosehips in a variety of bland or sweet foods.

Rose-mint tea

1 teaspoon dried petals
1/2 teaspoon dried mint
1 cup (250 ml) boiling water

Pour water over the herb, steep for 10 minutes, and strain. Enjoy!

Rose-petal sugar

1 part (by weight) dried rose petals
1 part (by weight) sugar

Pour into your blender or food processor and mix. Store in airtight jars in a dark place.

Rose-petal sugar adds flavor to desserts, whipped cream, cookies, and marzipan.

A simple rosehip soup

2 ounces (50 g) fresh cleaned rosehips
or 1 ounce (25 g) dried, soaked overnight
1 cup (250 ml) water
1 teaspoon potato starch
sugar

Simmer rosehips until they're soft, and then rub them through a sieve. Add potato starch and water. Bring to a boil. Add sugar to taste.

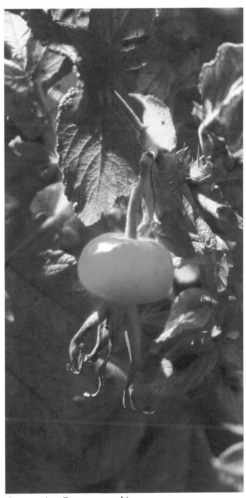

An overripe Rugosa rosehip.

OTHER USES

For weddings, gather lots of fresh rose petals, and sprinkle them over the bride. Spread them before the feet of a birthday child (or adult, as the case may be).

Add dried petals to potpourris, or use them in scented pouches.

Roses lose their scent rather too soon, so gather them afresh every year.

WARNINGS

Don't use sprayed roses—especially those from a florist, which contain insecticides, fungicides and vermicides. Even plant sellers may spray their offerings, so inquire before you buy.

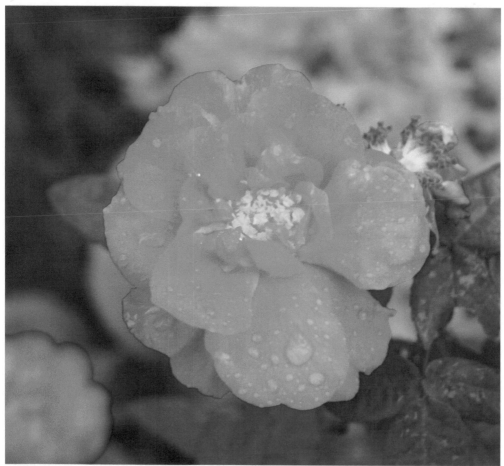

French rose (Rosa gallica) is among the most highly scented rose species.

ROSE BEADS

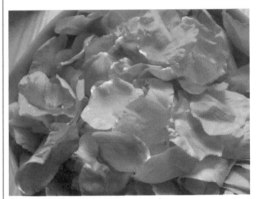

A bowl filled with fresh rose petals.

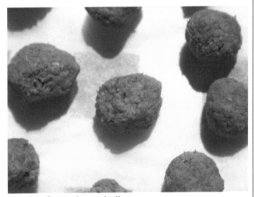

Freshly formed rose balls.

5–10 quarts (5–10 liters) tightly packed, strongly scented fresh rose petals
blender or food processor
a free week during which you may fiddle with roses (*mmm—lovely scent!*)
wire
dehydrator (optional)
small sewing needle
thread or fine floss

Fill a blender or food processor container about half-full of rose petals and pulse until they're the size of small crumbs. A few larger pieces won't matter, as long as there aren't too many. Repeat to process all your rose petals. If necessary, add a small amount of water.

Pour the chopped-up petals into a largish pan and add water to cover. Heat the mix to almost boiling, and then leave it at that heat for about an hour. Cool. Repeat the process once or twice a day for three to five days. Add water if the mass gets too dry.

Pour small batches (1/2 to 1 cup, or 125 to 250 ml) of the now-brownish mass into a piece of cloth, grab the corners, and wring.

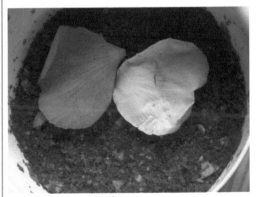

Straight from the blender.

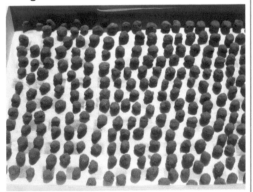

Balls formed from the rose mass.

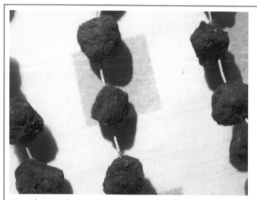

Dryish rose beads strung on wire.

Form small balls (1/3 inch or a centimeter across, say) from the dryish rose mass, and dry them on paper towels or clean cloth for a day or two, making sure they don't touch one another. This part can take a while, so be patient.

Cut steel wire in 5- to 8-inch (15–20 cm) lengths, and push the ends through your still-soft rose balls. One piece of wire will hold 10–20 beads.

Thicker wire will allow for a thicker threading needle later, but the thicker the wire, the more difficult it will be to keep the soft beads intact.

If you wire the beads too early, they'll fall apart. If you wait too long, they'll be too hard to work with.

Dry the beads on their wires for four or five days, or until they're dark, hard, and very dry. Or, if you don't want to wait that long, use a dehydrator on low heat.

Strip the beads from their wires. Pliers make quick work of this.

You needn't try to make your beads perfectly round and smooth. And don't coat the beads with anything; that eliminates the scent. There's no need to add rose essential oil or attar of roses.

Find a needle small enough to fit through the holes in your beads, and then thread them on string or floss. Or use beading wire.

The stronger a rose's scent, the more aromatic your beads will be.

Eight quarts or liters of tightly packed, fresh rose petals yields about 54 inches (or 150 cm) of strung rose beads.

Fresh beads release a strong and lovely scent of rose; older rose beads will release the scent when warmed in the hand.

If you store your beads in airtight containers between uses, they'll keep their scent for a century or more. Just think—your granddaughter might hold these in her hands one day!

Take out your rose beads when you're in need of some love, gentleness, courage—or a bit of prickliness.

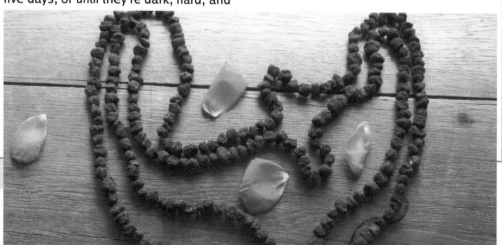

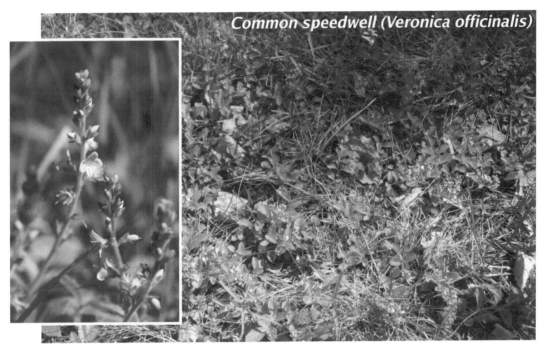

Common speedwell (Veronica officinalis)

SPEEDWELL

"In earlier times, when there were still witches, it was thought that speedwell could remove them."—Elias Lönnrot, Flora Fennica, *1866*

***Veronica* species:** Including common speedwell (*Veronica officinalis*), also called heath speedwell, common gypsyweed; germander speedwell (*Veronica chamaedrys*), also called angel's eyes, bird's-eye speedwell

Family: Plantain family, *Plantaginaceae* (*Scrophulariaceae*)

Perennial: Harvest in summer.

Habitat: Common speedwell grows along roadsides and forest paths. Germander speedwell is found in moist meadows and drainage ditches.

Appearance: Common speedwell is a delicate groundcover, with light blue to light purple small flowers on small upright flower heads.

Germander speedwell's largish, electric-blue flowers last for only a day, and turn downward in rain.

Important constituents: Tannins, bitters, resins, glycosides (aucubin), small amounts of essential oil

PICKING AND PROCESSING

Gather flowering plants or tops, remove yellowing leaves, and dry your take indoors out of the light. Cut the dried herb in 1-inch (2–3 cm) lengths, and store it in an airtight jar in a dark cupboard.

Common speedwell is much smaller than germander speedwell, and there's not a lot of it where it's found. If you go looking for this species, take a lot of patience with you.

Germander speedwell is more lavish in its growth, and harvesting it goes more quickly.

EFFECTS AND USES

Common and germander speedwell may be mild medicinal herbs, but they're versatile. They strengthen the liver, kidneys, digestion, and lungs. Don't expect wonders though—at least not immediately.

These speedwells are mildly astringent, and thus help with mild diarrhea.

The hot tea is good for coughs, asthma, and sore throat. It's been used for bronchitis, as well—but if you're suffering from bronchitis you should be sure to see a doctor, too.

Because common speedwell is bitter, it boosts the appetite and aids digestion. And common speedwell has been used to get liquids flowing more generally: the tea has been used to stimulate lactation, provoke sweating, as a diuretic, and to start menses flowing.

Used externally, speedwells are helpful for wounds, bruises, and small burns.

Speedwell tea

1 teaspoon dried common or germander speedwell
1 cup (250 ml) boiling water

Pour boiling water over the herb, steep for 10 minutes, and strain. Drink two to three cups a day.

FOOD USES

Add young speedwell shoots to salads, and use them as greens in salty foods.

Linnaeus thought common speedwell far better than black tea as a teatime drink. Germander speedwell is the less bitter, and tastes better to most people.

Speedwell salad

1 cup (250 ml) young shoots of common or germander speedwell
1 small yellow onion
2 hard-boiled eggs

Dressing:

1 tablespoon mustard
2 tablespoons vinegar
2 tablespoons olive oil
salt, pepper

Clean the shoots, chop the onion, and combine. Blend the dressing and add that to the salad. Decorate with sliced hard-boiled eggs.

Refrigerate for an hour, and serve.

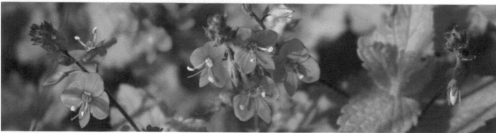

The lovely, bright blue flowers of germander speedwell (Veronica chamaedrys).

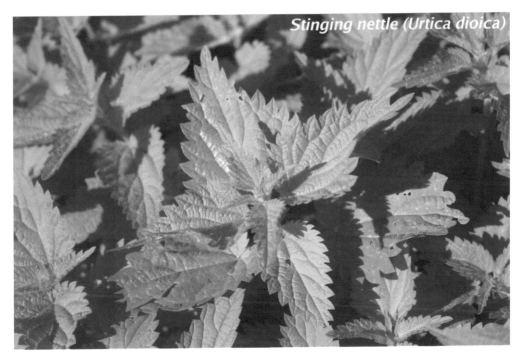

Stinging nettle (Urtica dioica)

STINGING NETTLE

It stings, it's one of our best wild greens, and it's a lovely medicinal plant.

Urtica dioica: Also called nettle and greater nettle.

Family: Nettle family, *Urticaceae*

Perennial: Harvest the young shoots in spring, the leaves and leafy tops in summer, and the seeds and roots in autumn.

Habitat: Stinging nettles are found in more or less lush places. Dwarf nettle (*Urtica urens*, also called dog nettle and lesser nettle), an annual with a fiercer sting and small roundish leaves, is often mistaken for its larger cousin.

You can use any reasonably gentle species of *Urtica* as you would stinging nettles.

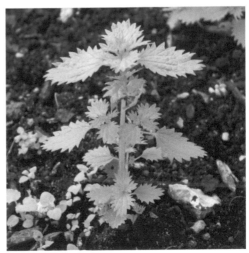

Dwarf nettle (Urtica urens).

Cultivation: Nettles propagate both by seeds and by underground runners.

I have seen nettles grow very nicely in rows like potatoes, so you can grow them in your garden, but I wouldn't plant it with herbs or flowers. It spreads almost as fast as true mints do and will sting you when you're weeding or picking herbs.

If you make nettle "fertilizer" from nettles in seed, you'll have young nettles spring up everywhere, even (if you used the fertilizer on them) in balcony boxes.

If you let stinging nettles grow with your black currants, you'll get more berries.

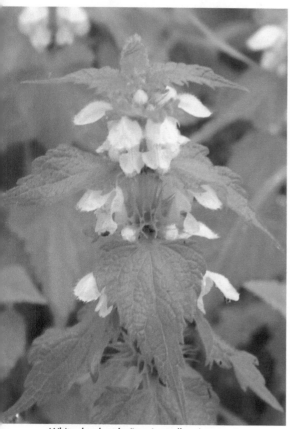

White deadnettle (Lamium album).

Look-alikes: A neighbor walking past my herb beds pointed to a catnip and said "Look, nettles!" He could have said the same of lemon balm, *Monarda*, or showy calamint; his eyes weren't trained to spot nettles.

In the wild, stinging nettles are easy to confuse with white deadnettle (*Lamium album*), which is quite similar when it's not in flower. When the two plants are in flower, though, they're easy to tell apart. Although white deadnettle has been used as a wild green and to stop bleeding, it's not stinging nettle.

Checking for the sting is a sure-fire way to distinguish nettles, but after checking a few dozen plants where some were nettles, you'll think all plants sting!

Important constituents: Large amounts of chlorophyll, fiber, flavonoids, tannins, plant acids and histamin, vitamins A, C, some Bs (green parts)

Nettle's mineral content is exceptional.

According to one study, 4 ounces (100 g) of fresh nettles contains 670 mg potassium, 590 mg calcium, 18 mcg chromium, 270 mcg copper, 86 mg magnesium, and 4.4 mg iron.

Another study gave the dried leaf 0.59–4.2 % calcium by weight, 0.35–3.7 % potassium, traces of chromium and copper, 0.17–0.86 % magnesium, and a trace to 0.2 % iron.

PICKING AND PROCESSING

Wear gloves for your nettle harvest, especially if you're picking a lot of it and don't want your fingers tingling into next week.

Don't pick nettles that grow near barns, heaps of manure, in pastures, or near an outhouse, if any of them have been in use during the preceding 12 months. Nettles in such spots may be lush, but they'll carry fecal bacteria.

Nettles growing on your compost or rich soil may contain large amounts of nitrates. The plants use them up in sunny weather, though, so pick them after three consecutive sunny days. In less lush spots, pick your nettles whenever you like.

Harvest **food nettles** in early summer. Gather the 8- to 12-inch (20–30 cm) shoots. You can continue picking whole shoots through the season, until the mature stems become too fibrous. Pick the green tops, then, instead, until the first flowers appear. To extend your wild greens season, cut the nettles as soon as they flower; they'll produce new shoots within four weeks.

For herbal uses, pick **whole shoots** from early summer until the plant starts to flower. Hang them to dry or use a dehydrator. Strip the dried leaves into glass jars and screw the lids on tightly.

Or powder the dried leaves and add to your green powder.

Leaves of flowering nettles have grown old on the stem and can contain calcium carbonate crystals that irritate the kidneys. Don't pick them. If your dish of nettles gives you a lower back pain, use

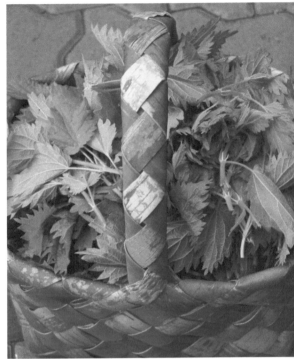

A basket of young nettle tops.

the rest of that batch for footbaths or fertilizer.

A few weeks after the plant flowers, the seeds ripen and become ready for harvest: the seed threads grow heavy and hang straight down along the stems. The best seeding nettles have long seed threads thick with seeds.

Pick **nettle seeds** with their stems and hang them to dry. You could harvest the seeds by stripping the stems, but you'll get large numbers of manylegged proteins doing that (and they won't necessarily find their way out of the nettle seeds you spread to dry).

Remove damaged or dead leaves before drying.

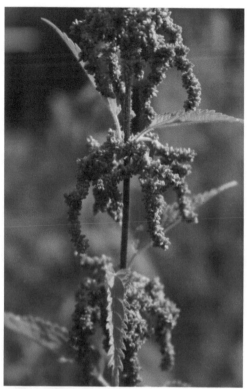
Nettle seed, ripe for picking.

Dig the bright yellow **roots** in late fall or early spring. Split any roots with diameters greater than 1/8 inch (3 mm) and remove beetle larvae and damaged areas. Dry them in a dehydrator, spread them to dry on clean cloth, or drape them over a string hung indoors out of the light.

EFFECTS AND USES

Stinging nettle is one of our best herbs for treating hay fever and similar allergic symptoms. Sensitivities or "allergies" are usually cumulative: there's pollen, you eat strawberries, and it's the last week before menses, so your body reacts with itchy mucosa, a runny nose, sneezing,

asthma, and so on. Use nettles regularly, though, and you can raise your tolerance for such irritants.

Those who suffer from hay fever should take nettle in any form from spring to fall. Some people with hay fever have been able to stop using pharmaceutical medications this way. (Those with asthma improve most by sticking to a dairy-free diet.)

If you're truly allergic to some substance, you'll become more sensitive to it with each exposure. For example, if those allergic to nickel don't avoid contact with the metal, eventually they will react even to coins and door handles.

Allergics should strengthen their livers: dandelion or chicory are good liver herbs. Those with low blood pressure should take a nondiuretic liver herb, instead—yellow dock root, for instance, or the root and lower stem bark of barberry *(Berberis* species).

The green parts of nettles in teas or as food are generally strengthening. Use them for mental or physical exhaustion. A mineral-rich nettle tea can speed recuperation from flu, surgery, or broken bones.

The leaves, shoots and young tops, and green seeds help in forming red blood cells for treating anemia.

The green parts are somewhat diuretic, help bolster the metabolism, and lower blood sugar somewhat. Because they strengthen both liver and kidneys, they help with some skin problems.

Externally, the sting of fresh nettles has been used to treat arthritic joint ailments. It enhances local blood supply, which helps reduce swelling and inflammation. (Bee and wasp stings have also been used in this way.)

Juiced nettles can help with joint pain, too. Take a tablespoon or two each day.

The root is diuretic and strengthens the bladder. A tea of nettle root helps with benign enlarged prostate.

Strengthen kidneys and adrenal glands with 1 or 2 teaspoons of the seeds every day. This helps with burnout, tiredness, exhaustion—and the resulting disappearing libido.

Some U.S. herbalists give a tincture of dried nettle seeds to people with kidney problems.

Using the seeds for exhaustion and tiredness is a traditional central European remedy: dishonest horse peddlers used to give a handful of nettle seed every day to their tired old nags for a few weeks before taking them to market. This gave them springy steps and shiny pelts, and they brought a handsome price. Because the new owner, in ignorance, didn't continue the nettle seed, the horses soon returned to their old tired selves.

In the early 20th century, a German naturopath used the trick in a home for the elderly. The residents got a tablespoon of nettle seeds each day. Sure enough, they got a spring in their step, a love of life—and a lovelife. (But, of course, they didn't turn into old nags when they stopped taking the nettle seed.)

Dried nettle seed helps with restlessness and poor concentration. Fresh seed, on the other hand, can aggravate restlessness in sensitive persons.

If you're generally sensitive, start with a pinch of the dried seed, or a few drops of a dried-seed tincture. If you don't generally react immediately to herbs, take teaspoons or tablespoons of the seed, as needed.

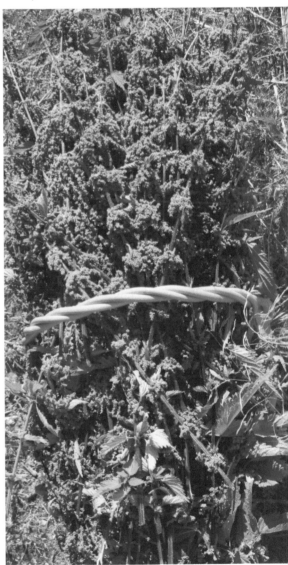

A basketful of nettles in seed.

A word about sex drive: if you do the cooking, the laundry, the cleaning, and keep track of the kids while your other half watches sport on the telly, a lack of libido isn't surprising. Get your partner to do the housework for a week or two, and you'll get it back. (Your mate might be too tired, though.) See to the basics before you start looking for magic pills or herbs.

Nettle tea

2–3 teaspoons dried nettle leaf, tops, or seed
1 cup (250 m) boiling water

Pour boiling water over the herb, steep for 10 minutes, strain. Drink two to three cups a day. If you live in a dry climate, add mallows.

Nettle decoction

2 teaspoons dried nettle leaf or tops
1 cup (250 ml) cold water

Add the herb and water to a pan, bring to a boil, steep for 12 to 15 minutes, and strain. Drink two to three cups a day. Again, add mallows if you live in a dry climate.

Nettle maceration

4–5 tablespoons dried nettle leaf or flowering tops
3 cups (750 ml) cold water

Pour water into a jar, add the herb, steep from 4 to 12 hours, and strain. Drink one to three cups a day. Add mallows if you live in a dry climate.

Nettle chai

4–5 teaspoons dried nettle leaf
1–2 cardamom pods
half a stick of cinnamon (optional)
1–3 cloves (optional)
3 cups (750 ml) boiling water

Pour water over the herb and spices, steep for 10 minutes, and strain. Enjoy with milk.

Add mallows if you live in a dry climate.

Nettle root decoction

1–2 teaspoons dried nettle root
1 cup (250 ml) cold water

Add the herb and water to a pan, bring to a boil, steep 12 to 15 minutes, and strain.

Drink one or two cups a day for benign prostatic overgrowth.

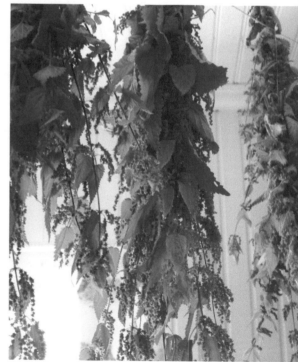

Nettles in seed, drying in bundles.

Juiced nettles

juicy young nettles

Cut the nettles into 1-inch (2–3 cm) lengths. Add them to your blender with a little water. Blend, strain.

Freeze in ice cube trays to use later, or use right away.

Take one or two tablespoons of nettle juice two to three times a day for a few weeks for exhaustion, tiredness, anemia, as a general strengthener, for hay fever and similar sensitivities, or for joint problems.

Nettle seeds

dried nettle seeds

Rub the seeds through a sieve. (If you don't, they'll still sting, and the mouth's membranes are far more sensitive than the skin of your fingers.)

Take a pinch to a tablespoon of nettle seed daily in thick liquids (such as yogurts and smoothies) or added to food at breakfast or lunch.

The seeds help with exhaustion, burnout, and tiredness.

Recuperative mineral tea

Pick those of the following herbs you can recognize easily:

1 part nettle
1 part horsetail
1 part red raspberry leaf
1 part green oats
1 part red clover
1 part lady's mantle

Dry the herbs separately or together, and store the blend in an airtight jar. Steep 1 teaspoon in 1 cup (250 ml) of boiling water for 5 to 10 minutes and strain. Drink three to four cups a day. This blend is excellent if you're recuperating from childbirth, surgery, broken bones, or flu.

Nettle seed tincture

4 ounces (100 g) dried seed
20 fluid ounces (500 ml) 120 proof grain alcohol (60 %)

Put the seed in a glass jar, cover with the alcohol, close tightly, and steep for two to four weeks. Strain, bottle, and label (example: "Nettle seed, 1:5 60 %, 08.2021, Hollow Woods").

Dosage is 15 to 20 drops, one to three times a day, for kidney problems, tiredness, and exhaustion, or one to three drops for restlessness, as needed.

FOOD USES

Soak fresh nettles in cold water for 10 minutes to encourage the manyleggeds to depart. Then lift small batches into boiling water. Within a few minutes the plants will be limp, the leaves a dark green, the stems a bright light green—and the sting will be gone.

Chop up the parboiled lot on a cutting board, or give them a whirl in your blender. The smaller they're cut, the smoother the texture, and the better the taste. (There's an unpleasant roughness to whole nettles.)

Use your nettles immediately, or freeze them in their cooking liquid.

Use nettles as you would spinach in a variety of salty foods, in stews, casseroles, omelets, bread, and in pastries.

Powdered dried nettles can be used as green powder by itself, or in a blend with other edible powdered greens. Add a spoonful to your meals.

You can also add powdered dried nettles to baked goods, omelets, and mashed potatoes.

Preserving

The best way to preserve nettles for food uses is to freeze the pre-boiled chopped greens. A large basketful of fresh nettles yields about 2 quarts (2 liters) of chopped-up nettles for the freezer.

Or, instead of chopping them, hang small bundles of boiled nettles to dry. Start the drying process outdoors until they've stopped dripping; then take them in to finish. Crush the thoroughly dried plants and store them in glass jars. Nettles dried this way taste completely different from regular dried nettles, but you can, of course, use either kind in your cooking.

OTHER USES

Mature stinging nettle is fibrous and can be processed as you would flax stems. The resulting thread is stronger than flax and is silk-like in appearance.

Nettle fertilizer

bucket of nettles

Cover the nettles with water. Let them stand for two weeks, stirring every few days. You'll end up with a smelly liquid and no discernible nettle parts (except perhaps for a few stems that might poke up above the mess—and seeds, which can germinate).

That liquid is your nettle fertilizer. Dilute 1:10—1 quart (liter) of nettle liquid to 10 quarts (liters) water. Pour it on the ground around plants as a fertilizer. It's too strong, even diluted, to be poured over the plants themselves.

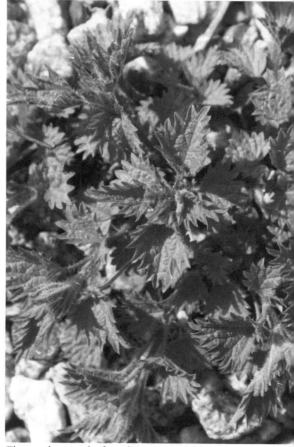

The regular growth of a solitary young nettle plant.

The bucket you use for this will stink to the heavens forever more, so don't use your best berry buckets for this. Use a disposable stirring stick, too.

Nettle compost starter

Pour diluted nettle fertilizer on dry compost.

(Urine does the trick, too. Here, I suggest the men of the household do their duty; the ladies can, of course, do it, too, but it's a tad more cumbersome for us.)

Nettle pest repellant

bucket of nettles

Cover the nettles with water and let them stand overnight. Pour the liquid over plants afflicted by soft-skinned pests, such as aphids.

Nettle hair conditioner

small bundle nettles
1 quart (liter) water

Boil the nettles for 10 to 15 minutes, strain, and cool. To use as a hair conditioner, pour the tea through your hair from 10 to 15 times. One pouring alone doesn't do much.

Warning: this can give a green tinge to light-colored hair.

A stinging nettle footbath

1 quart (liter) boiling water
fresh stinging nettles

Pick a small bundle of 6- to 8-inch (15–20 cm) nettle tops, cut them into 2-inch (5 cm) lengths, and drop them in boiling water. Return the water to a boil and simmer for five minutes, or until the nettles are limp.

Pour the water with the nettles into a bowl and dilute with cold water to a comfortable temperature. Keep shoes and a towel nearby, and enjoy your footbath for 10 to 20 minutes.

When you're done, throw the nettles with their cooled water under the nearest bush or onto the compost.

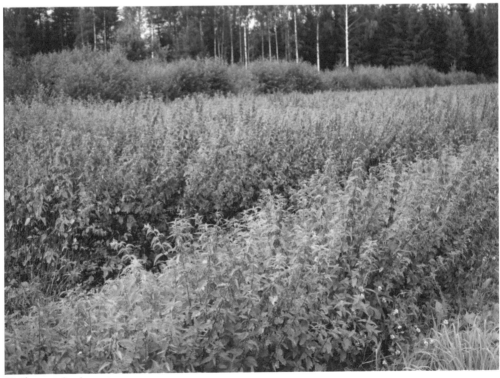

Nettles growing in rows.

WARNINGS

Carbonate crystals that form on older nettle leaves can irritate the kidneys. If you get a lower back pain from your nettles, stop ingesting that particular batch, and pick younger nettles in the future.

Nettles growing in very rich soil will be high in nitrates that become nitrites in our bodies—again, detrimental to health. Nettles use up these nitrates if they grow in the sun. You may pick such very lush nettles after a few days of sun exposure.

Nitrates can be high in some vegetables, such as spinach, green beans, red beets, and of course in commercially processed meats, such as cold cuts and sausages. Don't give such foods to infants younger than a year.

You'll find large stands of nettles near barns and outhouses and around pastures. Don't harvest these nettles if the structures have been in use during the preceding 12 months: fecal bacteria also thrive in those places.

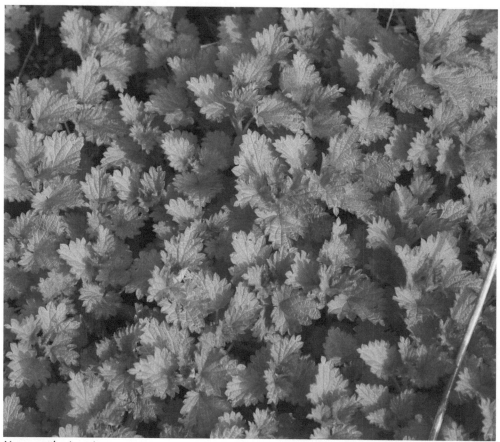

Young nettles in spring.

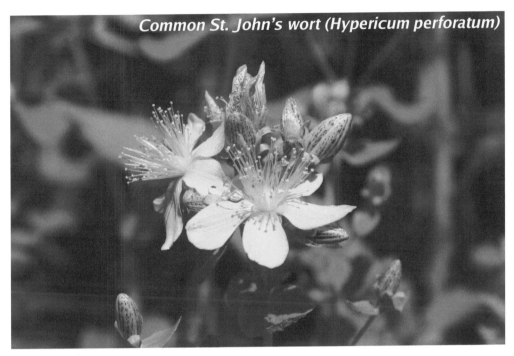

Common St. John's wort (Hypericum perforatum)

ST. JOHN'S WORT

A red color from yellow flowers? If that's not magic, I don't know what is.

***Hypericum* species:** Where I live we have two species in the wild—*Hypericum perforatum* (common St. John's wort, St. John's wort), and *Hypericum maculatum* (imperforate St. John's wort). You can use any species where the crushed flower or flower bud turns red.

Family: St. John's wort family, *Hypericaceae* (*Clusiaceae, Guttiferae*)

Perennial: Harvest at high summer.

Habitat: St. John's wort is common on dry meadows and roadsides.

Appearance: Because this plant grows to less than 18 inches (50 cm) tall, it can be tough to find among taller grasses.

Once you've spotted it, it's easy to confirm that it really is a St. John's wort: crush the flower. If it turns your fingers reddish purple, you're good to go.

In wet years the flower produces less of this color; you might get no color at all on a rainy summer's day. You also get less color in autumn.

You'll find the strongest St. John's wort on hot summer days at the height of a sunny summer. This is especially so at northern latitudes: the oil I extract from such a harvest turns a deep wine red, and I can't see through a dropperful of tincture.

Important constituents: Hypericin, hyperforin, resins, essential oil, bitters, tannins

These days it's believed the plant's hyperforin is behind its mood-lifting effects. Hypericin, once thought to be the active constituent, is now considered more detrimental than useful.

PICKING AND PROCESSING

Cut the upper 2–4 inches (5–10 cm) of the flowering tops when the plant starts to flower (mid-July here at northern latitudes; midsummer, perhaps, where you live).

The stems are tough, so use a knife or scissors or you'll pull up the whole flower stalk.

For depression, the St. John's wort's strongest part is its flower bud. For external uses, the strongest part is the seed pod. For both, the next best thing is the opened flower, and then the leaves and the stem.

When I gather St. John's wort, I don't care which species I have under my fingers, as long as it has the red color. I don't care, either, if it's mostly in flower, mostly in bud, or mostly in seed, as long as there is at least some yellow in the tops.

Drying St. John's wort

Use dried St. John's wort for teas or low-alcohol tinctures. Spread your take on old cotton sheets, or use a dehydrator set lower than 104 °F (40 °C). Because the seedpods of St. John's wort are large, it takes a long (long) time to dry the plant matter—at least three times longer than with other plants. Check by crushing a

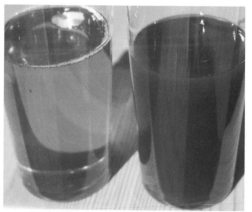
Infused oil from dried St. John's wort has little color. Oil from fresh herb can get so dark it's impossible to see through it, especially if sunlight falls onto it.

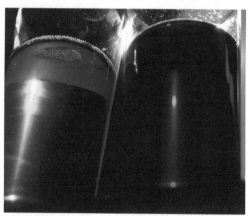
The same oils with the sun behind: oil from fresh herb is very dark.

few seedpods. Still moist inside? Keep on drying. Make absolutely sure the herb is dry before putting it into jars. Less-than-dry herb quickly gets moldy.

The St. John's wort you gather and dry yourself will lose its effect within a few years, so pick a lot during sunny summers. Purchased dried plant usually will be worthless within a year.

Herbal oil of St. John's wort

The infused oil must be made from the fresh plant, so either use it right after you pick it, or freeze the 1-inch (2–3 cm) pieces for infusing later. Because the oil is made from fresh herb, it must stand for a few days after straining to clear and settle out the water. Leave the oil in the sun as it clears; it turns turn a nice red within days. Oil infused from frozen St. John's wort works just as well and turns just as red in the sun, but it takes longer to clear than oil made from fresh herb.

Infused oil from dried St. John's wort takes months and months to turn red, and even then it won't be as deeply colored as the oil from fresh flowering tops.

The oil's redness is an indicator of its strength: the darker the better.

Tincture

Use either fresh herb or recently dried herb for tinctures.

EFFECTS AND USES

St. John's wort is a nerve plant. It's calming and reduces anxiety and depression, especially depression stemming from frustration. Your friends and loved ones will notice its cheering effect on you within three days of starting treatment. After a few weeks, you'll notice that you smile more and laugh at small mishaps instead of brooding over them.

This plant is good for mild to moderate depression. Although it has been shown to affect deep depression, this clinical level of disorder requires the help of a therapist or counselor, as well.

For Seasonal Affective Disorder (SAD—the depression you get in the darker months of the year), supplement St. John's wort with vitamins B, C, D, magnesium, zinc, iron, and fish oils.

St. John's wort is one of our best herbs for sleeplessness. Give it with either milky oats or California poppy. Tincture is best: keep the bottle on your bedside table, and you won't have to toss and turn for hours before finally getting up to make an insomnia tea.

Decades and centuries ago, St. John's wort was considered a liver and digestive herb. You can also use it as an anti-inflammatory. I've given powdered St. John's wort (*there's* a preparation that brings home the importance of properly drying the herb!) for chronic intestinal inflammations and as a tea or tincture in urinary tract infections.

Used externally, St. John's wort increases local blood supply and soothes inflammations. Use it for bruises, sprains, and swellings from trauma. Also try it for joint aches and pains, and for psoriasis. If it will work at all on an inflamed joint, it will reduce the swelling within 15 minutes. If this is the case, then use it

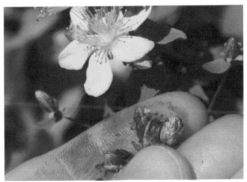

Yellow flowers, purple fingers.

often: you'll find it works every time, and your joints can heal now that their blood supply isn't strangled.

St. John's wort helps heal small wounds and can reduce recently formed scars. It's also useful for nerve damage: if the nerves on one side of a scar send a different signal from those on the other side, they're misconnected. Rub St. John's wort on the spot daily for a few weeks or months, and the problem should clear up.

St. John's wort tincture

From fresh herb:

4 ounces (100 g) fresh flowering tops, cut in 1/3–1-inch (1–3 cm) pieces
8 fluid ounces (200 ml) 190 proof grain alcohol (95 %)

From dried herb:

4 ounces (100 g) dried flowering tops, cut in 1/3–1-inch (1–3 cm) pieces
20 fluid ounces (500 ml) 120 proof grain alcohol (60 %)

Put the pieces into a glass jar, cover with the alcohol, and close the lid tightly. Steep for two to four weeks. Then strain, bottle, and label (example: "SJW, 1:5 60 %, 09.2021, Grandma's garden").

The dose is 5–30 drops, one to three times a day.

Again, the deeper the color, the stronger the tincture.

St. John's wort tea

1–2 teaspoons St. John's wort dried or fresh flowering tops
1 cup (250 ml) boiling water

Pour boiling water over the herb. Steep for 10 minutes, and strain. Drink up to three cups a day. The redder the tea, the

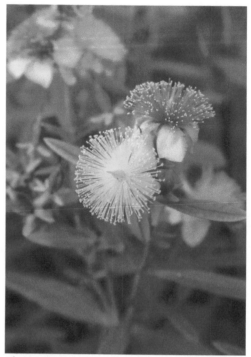

The gorgeous Kalm's St. John's wort (Hypericum kalmianum) won't work: neither the flowers nor the flower buds color anything red.

stronger it is.

Oil and salve of St. John's wort

Make an herbal oil from the fresh herb (page 18), and then make a salve from the oil (page 22).

WARNINGS

The single constituent hypericin is a mono amine oxidase inhibitor (MAOI). If you take hypericin alone, you must avoid chocolate, red wine, and some cheeses—the same foods everyone avoids who uses MAOI drugs.

However, teas, tinctures, and powders made from the flowering tops of the St. John's wort plant are negligible MAOIs.

Don't worry about these foods when using them.

Hypericin taken internally as a single constituent causes sensitive people to sunburn easily.

Grazing on the whole plant can give animals such as sheep and horses severe sunburn, especially in their hides' unpigmented areas. A white mouth with sunburn blisters can cause livestock to stop eating. But these grazers ingest a lot more St. John's wort than we ever could.

If you take blood-thinning pharmaceutical drugs, introduce new foods and herbs carefully, and ask your doctor to monitor your clotting factor closely.

I don't recommend herbs to people who take drugs to stop organ transplant rejections. (And I don't quite understand why St. John's wort issues with transplant patients are trotted out anytime the herb is mentioned to docs.)

St. John's wort can aggravate the side effects of pharmaceutical depression drugs. Avoid using both at the same time.

The notion that St. John's wort reduces the effectiveness of the contraceptive pill is theoretical. St. John's wort will enhance the liver's CYP450 enzyme, but this enhancement is not strong enough for practical implications. A forgotten pill or bout of diarrhea are far more likely to result in an unwanted pregnancy.

If you've been taking St. John's wort for depression, and it's time to end the course of treatment, wean yourself from the herb gradually. Although it's not dangerous to stop cold-turkey, you may startle those around you with your three days' temper.

OTHER USES

Although infused oil of St. John's wort makes a respectable sunscreen (with a strength of about 11), using the herb internally can make some people more susceptible to sunburn.

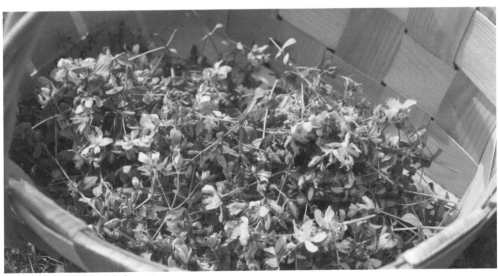

Flowering tops of St. John's wort.

EARACHE

These days olive and almond oils are available to buy anywhere, but there was a time when you could buy them only from a pharmacy—for earache.

But any bog-standard cold-pressed food oil will help with earaches. Put two to five drops into the achy ear, and wait for the pain to stop.

Of course, if the eardrum has a hole in it, you can't do that. In that case, massage some oil behind the ear. That works, too, if more slowly.

A more effective earache oil is infused with mullein (*Verbascum* species); any mullein will work.

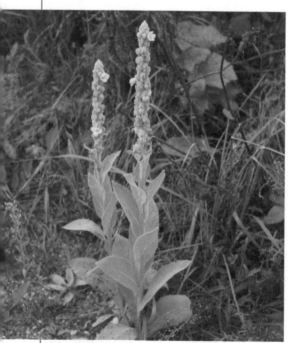

*Great mullein (*Verbascum thapsus*) in flower.*

I usually lop off flower stalks, although most herb books will tell you that you should only pick single flowers. Dry the flowers (or the flower stalks) in a shady spot indoors for a week or 10 days, or until they're really dry. Store them in an airtight glass jar in a dark cupboard. Use them within a year or two.

Mullein ear oil

1/2–1 cup (100–250 ml) cold-pressed oil
mullein flowers
or flower stalks cut into 1-inch (2–3 cm) lengths

Pour the oil into a stainless steel bowl (or upper part of a double-boiler) and add mullein flowers; the oil should just cover them. Place the bowl over a waterbath for two to three hours. Strain the oil through a coffee filter and bottle.

Use from two to five drops per achy ear (adult), one or two drops (children).

Mullein reduces both inflammation and pain, so it's ideal for earaches. And because both oil and mullein are nontoxic, you can add another few drops every hour or so, as needed.

The reason for kids' earaches is almost always too much mucus in the ears. That again stems from mucus-producing foods, such as dairy, white flour, and refined sugar. The problem often clears up once these foods are reduced or removed from the diet.

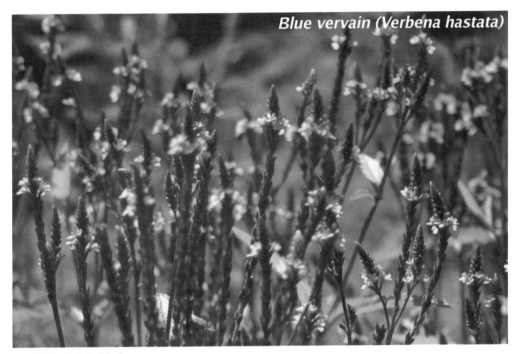

Blue vervain (Verbena hastata)

VERVAIN

Vervain might have become the herb for depression—if St. John's wort hadn't gotten there first.

Vervain (**Verbena species**) and mock vervain (**Glandularia species**): Annuals include

- Purpletop vervain (*Verbena bonariensis*), also called clustertop vervain and tall verbena
- Dakota mock vervain (*Glandularia bipannitifida*), also called prairie verbena
- Garden verbena (*Glandularia x hybrida*), also called florist's verbena
- Rose mock vervain (*Glandularia canadensis*), also called rose verbena

Perennials include

- Common vervain (*Verbena officinalis*), also called vervain, herb of the cross
- Blue vervain (*Verbena hastata*), also called swamp verbena, American vervain

Family: Vervain family, *Verbenaceae*

Annual/Perennial: Generally, upright species with ax-like flowering tops survive hard winters, while those with showier flowers are grown as annuals.

Harvest any of them from summer to fall.

Cultivation: For herbal use, it's best to grow annual species from seed; you'll find it next to impossible to find summer flower vervain plants grown without pesticides.

You can grow the perennials from seed or buy plants.

Vervains and mock vervains require full sun and well-drained soil. The perennials sometimes self-seed; I move stray seedlings nearer their parent plants, both for showiness and to make an easier harvest.

Appearance: Mock vervains are usually creeping or trailing, with large, showy flower heads. Colors range from white and pink through dark purple. Some plants have several colors in a single flower head.

Common vervain is noticeable only if grown in a largish cluster; its tiny flowers are otherwise next to invisible on their long stalks.

Flower heads of blue vervain are denser and larger and can be showy when grouped.

Both perennials can reach a height of about 36 inches (1 m). Purpletop vervain's showy flowers can reach 5 feet (1.5 m).

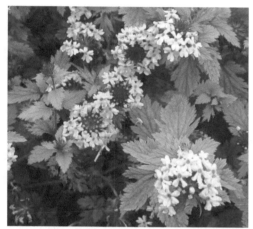

Rose mock vervain (Glandularia canadensis) *in flower.*

Important constituents:
Polysaccharides (stachyose 1.3 %), phenolic acids (caffeic acid 1 %), glycosides (verbenalin 0.3–0.5 %, aucubin, verbenin)

PICKING AND PROCESSING

Collect the flowering tops from midsummer to late autumn. Remove yellowing and dead leaves and dead flower heads.

Dry the herb and cut it into 1-inch (2–3 cm) lengths. Store in an airtight jar out of the light.

EFFECTS AND USES

Vervains relax. They're good for tense or over-amped bodies and minds.

They allow you to let go of unrealistic expectations, which makes the vervains great for relieving many kinds of stress. Try a vervain or mock vervain tea or tincture if these unrealistic expectations result in depression, frustration, exhaustion, or sleeplessness, or if they cause headaches or stiff necks.

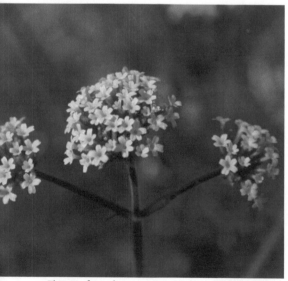

Flower of purpletop vervain (Verbena bonariensis).

Because these plants are bitter, they can aid digestion (if you let the bitter taste touch your taste buds).

The vervains have been helpful for menstrual and digestive cramps, coughs, and asthma.

A hot vervain tea helps you sweat.

Don't go overboard with vervain if you haven't used the plant before. Too large a dose can nausate you. Tolerance is individual: where even one cup of the tea can be too much for one person, another can drink it by the quart with no problem.

Vervain tincture

From fresh herb:

4 ounces (100 g) fresh herb in 1/3–1-inch (1–3 cm) lengths
8 fluid ounces (200 ml) 190 proof grain alcohol (95 %)

From dried herb:

4 ounces (100 g) dried herb in 1/3–1-inch (1–3 cm) lengths
20 fluid ounces (2 cups, or 500 ml) 100 proof grain alcohol (50 %)

Put the herb in a glass jar, cover with alcohol, and close the lid tightly, and steep two to four weeks. Strain, bottle, and label (example, fresh: "Blue vervain, 1:2 95 %, 07.2021, my garden"; example, dried: "Vervain, 1:5 50 %, 10.2021, the front yard").

Dosage is one to three drops as needed for stress, depression, and/or tense, achy neck or muscles.

Sometimes a tincture of fresh vervain will turn into globs. If the bottle is shaken, the globs break up into tiny gel-like droplets. The gel or globs won't affect the tincture's effectiveness.

If you feel nauseated after a few drops of

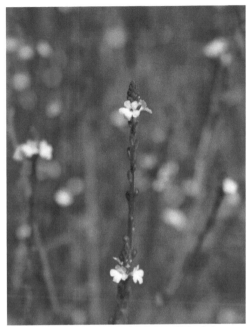

*Flower of common vervain (*Verbena officinalis*).*

vervain tincture, you've exceeded your threshold. Use smaller amounts less often. Try adding a drop to a glass of water and taking a tablespoonful of that, instead.

Vervain tea

1 teaspoon dried or fresh vervain
8 ounces (250 ml) boiling water

Pour boiling water over the herb, let steep for 10 minutes, and strain. Sip the tea. If you feel nauseated, you've exceeded your tolerance for vervain. Drink smaller amounts more seldom in the future.

WARNINGS

Avoid vervains if you're pregnant or lactating.

Too large a dose can cause nausea.

ITCHING

Once you've determined your itch doesn't indicate anything serious, try one of the following remedies.

- The juice of chickweed (*Stellaria media*) gives immediate relief from mosquito bites or nettle sting. You'll usually find chickweed in moist rich soil. It can be so juicy you can rub a handful into a ball and squeeze a few drops of juice from it with one hand. Drop the juice straight onto the itching spot. Or take a handful of fresh chickweed, rub it between your hands, and massage the now-moist herb on itchy skin.

- The transparent gel that forms at the base of the leaves of green and growing *Rumex* species (docks) is also effective against itches. It's most abundant where the plants grow in damp spots, but rainy weather increases this gel in docks growing even in sand. (After you've applied it you'll have gel on your hands, so make sure you're near a place where you can wash them.)

- Juice from various species of balsam or jewelweed (*Impatiens* species) work for itch, as well. It's most abundant in thick stems. Pluck a plant, crush the stem, and rub the juice over itchy skin. (Some jewelweeds have an awful smell. If your local species is one of these, after you apply it you'll want to wash your hands sooner rather than later.)

- Some regular rolled oats added to a bath soothes a full-body itch. Spread a square of cheesecloth (about 15 inches or 40 cm on a side), pour a cup of oats in the center, gather the the corners to make a pouch, and then bind the pouch with a bit of string. Make sure no oats can escape.

As you run your bath let tepid water run through the oats pouch, and then get in to enjoy your bath. As you bathe, gently press or rub the pouch on your itchy skin. If the cheesecloth is too rough, mix rolled oats with just enough water to make a thick paste and spread that on affected areas.

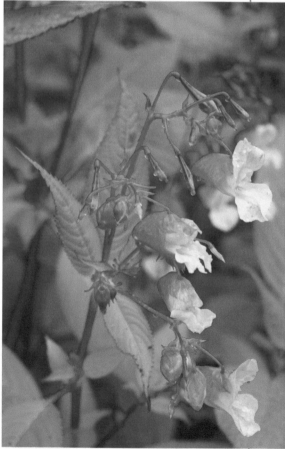

*Flowering tops of Indian balsam (*Impatiens glandulifera*).*

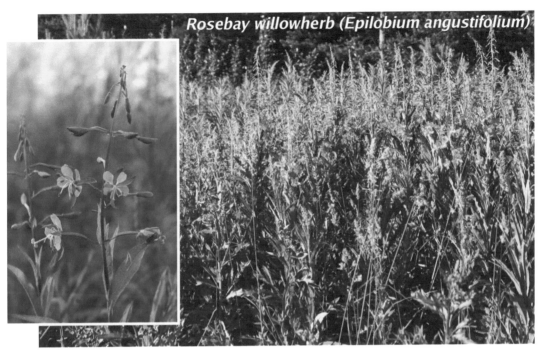

Rosebay willowherb (Epilobium angustifolium)

ROSEBAY WILLOWHERB

A useful beauty.

Epilobium angustifolium
(*Chamaenerion angustifolium*): Also called fireweed.

Family: Evening primrose family, *Onagraceae* (*Oenotheraceae*)

Perennial: Harvest in summer.

Habitat: Rosebay willowherb is common along roadsides, in meadows, and at forest edges. It spreads by both seed and runners and often covers large areas.

Appearance: The young shoots have an abundance of tiny leaves at the top; they are hairless. Any leaves on the stem spiral up along it. The leaves have smooth edges.

The flowering plant turns whole landscapes bright purple.

Look-alikes: Yellow and tufted loosestrife (*Lysimachia vulgaris, L. thyrsiflora*)—the loosestrifes have opposite leaves; narrowleaf hawkweed (*Hieracium umbellatum*)—which has toothed leaf edges.

Important constituents: Tannins, protein, vitamin C, carotene, trace minerals, a hint of mucilage

129

PICKING AND PROCESSING

Use only the leaves. Gather them before the plant flowers: take a firm grip of the stem and yank it up. Then you can either take the stems home with you or strip the leaves into your basket. Stems in leaf can be hung to dry in small bundles.

Rosebay willowherb stalks are considerably larger and heavier than those of other herbs. If you dry the herb in bundles, make sure the twine you use is strong, and that the nail or hook is sturdy and attached to a stud or rafter, not just drywall.

Dry the leaf separately from flowers or flower buds. The dried seedpods (found with small flower buds) burst at the lightest touch and fill the area with white fluff to the point that you can't breathe. If you choose to keep your fluffy willowherb leaf, you'll get a tiny fluff explosion every time you open the jar. It's better to pick and dry new willowherb without flowers or flower buds.

The dried flowers lend a splash of color to dried tea blends. Pick them without their stems.

You can use any willowherb like rosebay willowherb. If I had to choose another species, I'd prefer one as large and as easy to gather.

Primrose leaf (*Oenothera* species) can be used in place of fireweed.

EFFECTS AND USES

Fireweed leaf is good for gut mucosa. I use it as a base in tea blends for digestive trouble.

The leaf also treats benign enlarged prostate. For that, I recommend daily walks in addition to herbs; the walks will enhance blood supply to the area.

Fireweed was used for centuries to remedy the "green diarrhea" resulting from the change from winter foods (salted meat and fish, canned vegetables) to spring's first fresh produce. Because it enhances general enzyme production in the stomach lining and pancreas, the tea is still helpful for preventing the upset gut that comes with dietary changes.

Take willowherb tea regularly, and you'll find it easier to digest the foods you eat only now and then. Drink it if you plan, for example, to change your diet from omnivore to vegetarian, or vice versa. Drink it before you go abroad, too, to keep traveler's diarrhea at bay.

Use a strong willowherb tea as a gargle for inflammations in the mouth and throat.

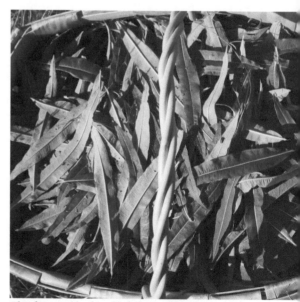

This fireweed leaf is of a fairly good quality, although it's harvested in late summer.

Willowherb tea

1–2 teaspoons dried or fresh willowherb
leaves
1 cup (250 ml) boiling water

Pour water over the herb, steep for 10
minutes, and strain. Drink up to three
cups a day.

FOOD USES

The very young shoots of willowherb can
be used like a kind of wild asparagus.
Remove and discard the tuft of leaves at
the top, cook the shoots as you would
any asparagus, and serve with a nice
sauce or aioli.

You can add the discarded tops to your
herbal tea, or to stews and soups.

The young leaves make a nice addition to
stews and salads.

During the world wars, Europeans used
fermented willowherb leaf in place of
scarce Chinese tea. In Russia, fermented
willowherb leaf was sold under the name
of "Kaporie Tea." (See page 14 for more
on fermentation.)

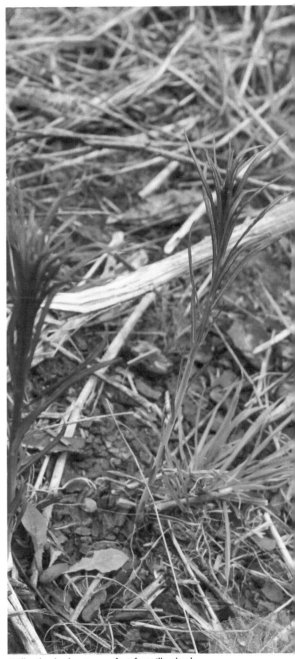

*Willowherb shoots, perfect for willowherb
asparagus.*

BLEEDING

Shepherd's purse (*Capsella bursa-pastoris*) makes an efficient styptic. I've used it for small wounds on the hands or face—they usually bleed profusely—and in heavy menses. You can also use it for nosebleeds.

Show deeper wounds to a doctor. (Of course, you should always see a doctor if you have internal bleeding!)

Shepherd's purse is a common weed in dry places. Pay close attention, though: its heart-shaped seedpods resemble those of penny-cresses (*Thlaspi* species). Penny-cresses aren't toxic, but they won't stop bleeding. Look carefully

*Seedpods of shepherd's purse (*Capsella bursa-pastoris*).*

and the difference becomes plain: seeds of shepherd's purse have straight edges and are of uniform thickness; penny-cress seeds are thicker in the middle, with flaring rounded "wings" on the edges. Also, shepherd's purse tastes of cabbage, while penny-cresses are more oniony.

Dried shepherd's purse has a limited shelf-life. The tincture lasts longer.

In summertime it's easy enough to pick a fresh leaf, crush it between your fingers, and apply it to a bleeding spot. Dry or tincture the herb to use the rest of the year.

For nosebleed, eat a leaf or take a few drops of tincture every few minutes until the bleeding stops. Or drink a cup of shepherd's purse tea.

The tea or tincture helps with heavy menses, too. Use for a few days before menses and during bleeding. (And make sure you get enough magnesium, iron, and vitamins B and C.)

Shepherd's purse doesn't keep for long, so harvest new herb every year.

If you can't find shepherd's purse, try yarrow, cayenne pepper, usnea, or white deadnettle.

Tea of shepherd's purse

1–2 teaspoons dried or fresh shepherd's purse
1 cup (250 ml) boiling water

Pour water over the herb, steep for 5 to 10 minutes, and strain. Drink two to three cups a day.

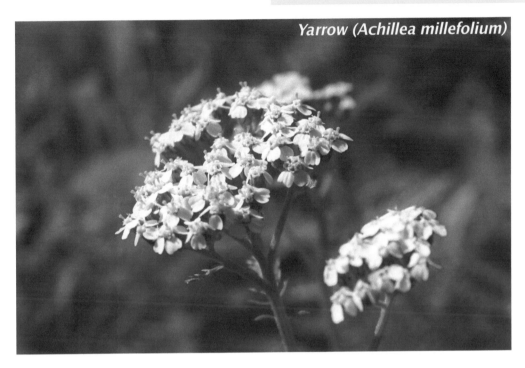

Yarrow (Achillea millefolium)

YARROW

Wherever it grows, yarrow has been used for everything that ails humankind.

Achillea millefolium: Also called milfoil, thousand leaf, woundwort

Family: Daisy family, *Asteraceae* (*Compositae: Tubuliflorae*)

Perennial: Harvest in summer.

Habitat: Yarrow can be found in meadows and wastelands, ditches and lawns.

Cultivation: Yarrow requires loose soil and at least part-time sun.

Appearance: Leaves are dark green and divided. The Latin millefolium means "a thousand leaves." Flowers of wild yarrows are white or sometimes pink. Garden varieties and species boast a full range of color, from brilliant golds to deep reds and lavenders.

Look-alikes: The leaves of yarrow resemble those of a number of plants, including caraway and carrot. The flowers of sneezewort (*Achillea ptarmica*) are larger than those of yarrow.

Important constituents: Essential oils, bitters, alkaloids, tannins, inulin (not insulin), flavonoids, plant acids

PICKING AND PROCESSING

Cut the flowering tops in high summer, either just under the flower head or with a generous length of stem.

133

If you can still see yellow stamens, the flowers are in their prime. Grayish flowers have lost some effect. Leave the brownish ones to seed.

Dry the blooms you cut with their stems in hanging bundles; dry the cut flower heads spread on a cotton bedsheet or large cloth. If you didn't get to the flowers in time, pick and dry the leaves, instead; they're effective, too, although less powerful than the flowers.

Dried yarrow remains useful for two or three years. The flavor of older yarrow gets milder and milder as it ages.

Dig the roots in loose soil, such as gravel or sand. Get a good grip of the plant's base, wiggle it as you pull upward, and you'll have a small pile of little roots in no time. Keep only the most substantial rootlets, cut them in 2-inch (5 cm) lengths, and let them dry thoroughly. Store dried root bits in an airtight glass jar. They'll stay good for two years, tops, so gather new roots every year.

Yarrow is in the daisy family. If you're allergic to mugwort or ragweed, you can get allergic symptoms from yarrow, too.

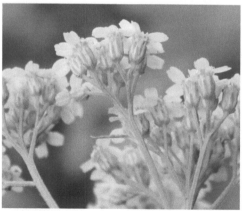
Yarrow flowers seen from underneath.

EFFECTS AND USES

Yarrow is useful for just about anything:

Skin and hair. Because yarrow makes the skin secrete more, it's especially helpful for dry skin. This is part of yarrow's liver-strengthening effect. Strengthening the liver helps with fat digestion, which can be seen as more fat getting to the skin, if the skin was dry to start with.

A bath of yarrow remedies a variety of skin problems. Use the lukewarm tea as a wash for acne.

Yarrow also helps dissolve scars.

I've heard that yarrow will even make your hair grow. For this, you should rub the decoction into your hair every day. (Note that a possible reason for hair loss, especially in women, is an underactive thyroid. Don't take an herb for the symptom; instead, find out the cause and remedy that.)

Lungs. Inhale the steam of a hot yarrow tea for respiratory tract problems—and then drink it!

Digestion. As a bitter, yarrow strengthens the digestion, starting with saliva secretion. It also stimulates secretions of stomach, gallbladder, pancreas and intestines.

Use yarrow to curb overeating as well.

For hemorrhoids, take a yarrow bath, or wash the area with cooled yarrow tea, or drink three to four cups of tea a day for a few weeks. Do other things, too, of course: move your buttocks, go for a walk, do scissor-leg movements—do your best to enhance the blood circulation in the area. Men will be happy to hear that a good long walk two to three times a week, coupled with leg-scissors exercises, will help eliminate hemorrhoids and enhance their erections.

Immune system. Yarrow works a little like echinacea, in that it makes the white blood cells more "trigger-happy." A hot yarrow tea makes you sweat, which can be helpful in stuck fevers. If you don't like the tea, you can take the tincture in hot water.

Yarrow's essential oils help the body rid itself of pathogens.

Ladies' problems. Because yarrow strengthens the liver, the hormones are better organized, and this leads to fewer problems with menses, among other things.

Yarrow stops bleeding, and is therefore helpful with heavy menses. The essential oils help relieve menstrual cramps. The tea is dependable for leucorrhea.

The urinary tract. Yarrow stimulates the kidneys somewhat. It's also helpful in urinary tract infections (UTIs), especially if they're long-term. Here it's the sum of its actions that help: it's astringent, it's styptic, it's diuretic, and it's aromatic. For long-term UTIs I recommend also removing sugar from the diet. It's also a good idea to take cranberry or lingonberry juice, one or the other mallow, and lactobacilli daily for a few weeks. Shepherd's purse, calendula, and St. John's wort also help strengthen and heal the damaged mucous membrane.

Give yarrow to bedwetting or incontinent children.

The liver. Milk thistle (*Silybum marianum*) helps regenerate damaged liver tissue. Yarrow works a little bit like that, although it's considerably weaker.

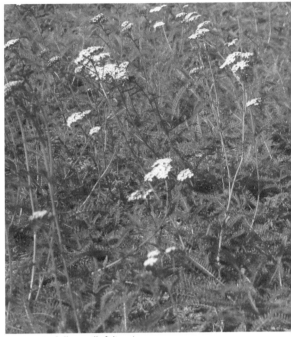

Yarrow (Achillea millefolium).

The musculoskeletal system. Take advantage of yarrow's circulatory enhancement, and use it externally (as salves, oils, baths etc.) or internally (as tea, decoction, tincture) for joint pain, muscle aches, and bruises.

The lymph system. Take the tea or tincture in small, regular amounts for wounds, or apply freshly crushed flowers or leaves to them.

The circulatory system. Yarrow is a good styptic. Use it in nosebleeds, on small wounds in the face or hands, for heavy menses, and so on.

Regular use of yarrow helps lower high blood pressure by enhancing digestion and strengthening the kidneys and liver. Thus, it won't lower an already low blood pressure.

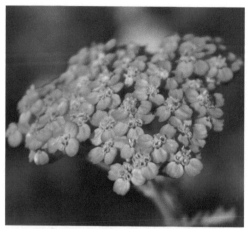

Use pink-flowering yarrow just as you would the white.

Other uses. The tannins in yarrow make it astringent. That's why it's good for diarrhea, sunburned skin, and inflamed gums.

Also, chewing the recently dried root can relieve toothaches.

Oil and salve of yarrow

Make an herbal oil from the dried herb (page 18), and then make a salve from the oil (page 22).

Use it on joint pain, hemorrhoids, varicosities, bruises, and eczema.

Yarrow tea

1–2 teaspoons dried yarrow
1 cup (250 ml) boiling water

Pour boiling water over the herb, steep for 10 minutes, and strain. Drink up to three cups a day for digestive upset, menstrual problems, heavy menses, and mild respiratory tract problems.

Use the cooled tea as a gargle if you have halitosis and as a wash for wounds and eczemas.

A fever tea for kids

1 teaspoon dried yarrow
1 teaspoon dried chamomile
pinch of aniseed or fennel seed
1 cup (250 ml) boiling water

Pour boiling water over the herb, steep for 5 minutes, and strain. Let the child sip the tea until she either feels better or falls asleep.

A yarrow bath

2–3 handfuls dried yarrow
1 quart (liter) water

Put the herb and the water into a pan. Bring to a boil; then turn off heat and steep for 10 minutes. Strain and pour into bathwater. Add enough cold water to make a comfortable bath. Get in and enjoy!

Yarrow tincture

From fresh flowers:

4 ounces (100 g) fresh flowers
8 fluid ounces (200 ml) 190 proof grain alcohol (95 %)

From dried flowers:

4 ounces (100 g) dried flowers
20 fluid ounces (500 ml) 100 proof grain alcohol (50 %)

Put the flowers into a glass jar, cover with the alcohol, and close the lid tightly. Steep for two to four weeks. Then strain, bottle, and label (example, from fresh material: "Yarrow, 1:2 95 %, 07.2021, the forest meadow"; example, from dried: "Yarrow, 1:5 50 %, 12.2021, picked on the downs").

Dosage is 10–30 drops, one to three times a day.

Yarrow decoction

2 teaspoons dried yarrow
1 cup (250 ml) cold water

Add the herb and water to a pan, bring to a boil, simmer for 5 minutes, and strain.

FOOD USES

Add young yarrow leaves to salads, soups, stews, and herbal sandwich spreads.

To use larger amounts in your cooking, first parboil the leaves and discard the water to tame the flavor a bit.

OTHER USES

Yarrow has been used instead of hops in beers.

Yarrow stalks are a traditional way to divine using the *I Ching*. For that, you need 50 equally long, similarly thick flower stalks. When you gather your own set, pick a bit more than the 50 so you'll have some spares.

WARNINGS

If you're sensitive to yarrow, handling it may give you a skin rash. Furthermore, allergies to mugwort or ragweed can mean you're sensitive to yarrow, as well. If you find you're sensitive to yarrow, by all means stop using it.

Sometimes yarrow can turn your urine brown; it's not dangerous.

Don't consume large amounts of yarrow if you are pregnant.

Too much yarrow can give you a headache or make you dizzy. If that happens, use common sense and take smaller amounts of the plant, or stop using it altogether.

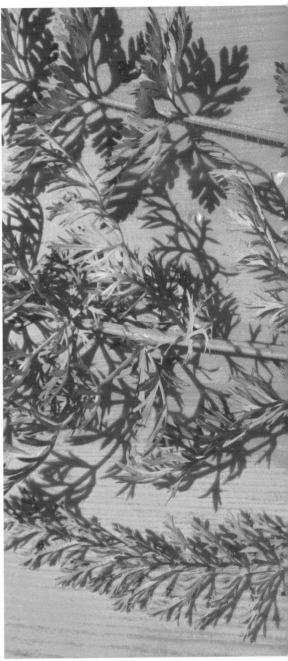

Top to bottom: leaves of carrot, caraway, and yarrow.

TOOTHACHE

When you have an achy tooth, yarrow root is the best herbal help you can get. Take a 2-inch (5 cm) piece of stout rootlet, chew it for a bit, place it between the cheek and gum on the painful side, and keep it there for about 15 minutes.

Spit out the root when the pain stops. If the pain returns, repeat with another piece of root.

Because you will usually get a toothache on Friday night, when it's impossible to get an appointment with the dentist, plan on having enough root pieces to make it over a weekend.

I've found that 20–30 pieces per toothache is a nice amount. You can, of course, harvest more than that.

The roots lie close to the soil surface and usually are only 4–8 inches (10–20 cm) long. You'll harvest them most easily from yarrows growing in gravel or loose sandy soil.

Use the brown, older roots (or, better, underground runners) for toothache, not the reddish or greenish younger ones.

To dry the roots for winter use, spread them on a paper towel or cotton cloth or old sheet and leave them for a week or 10 days—until they're dry enough to break instead of bend.

Store the dried roots in airtight jars. They'll keep for two years.

A toothache can be a sign of infection under an old filling or in a root canal, so try to see a dentist if you have a toothache. These hidden bacteria already have sidestepped your defenses. If they move out, they can move in on your heart or kidneys.

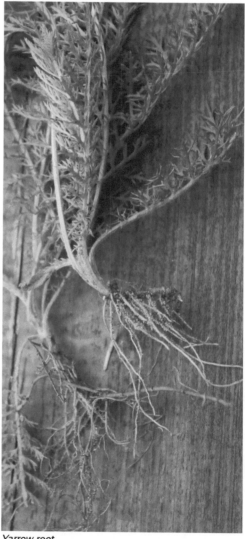

Yarrow root.

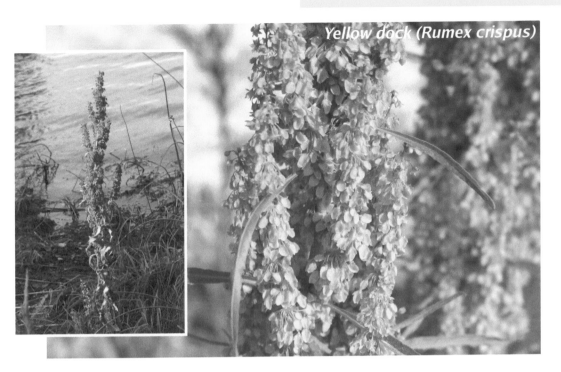

Yellow dock (Rumex crispus)

YELLOW DOCK

The yellower the root, the stronger it is.

Rumex species: The tap-rooted docks

Family: Knotweed or smartweed family (*Polygonaceae*)

Perennial: Harvest from summer to fall.

Habitat: Docks are common weeds just about everywhere.

Appearance: Rumex species include both docks and sorrels. Docks have tap roots and large green to greenish-red flower clusters. When the seeds mature they turn a deep reddish brown; the seed heads retain their seeds through most of the winter.

Sorrels, on the other hand, have delicate stems, small flower clusters, and "runners"—roots that run above and a little way under the ground, generating new plants here and there.

Important constituents: Tannins, 3–4 % antraquinone glycosides.

Color indicates root strength: the deeper the yellow, the more active constituents, and so the smaller the needed dose.

PICKING AND PROCESSING

Dock roots are at their best in the fall, but you can dig them whenever the ground isn't frozen.

Rinse the roots and slice them a quarter-inch thick or so (5 mm), or into matchsticks a quarter-inch by an inch-and-a-half (5 mm by 4 cm). Dry them on an old bedsheet or other clean cotton cloth, or use a dehydrator.

Dehydrator-dried roots retain some of their surface yellow; slower drying makes for deep reddish-brown roots.

Unfortunately, the yellow of dehydrator-dried roots isn't so pronounced that you can tell how yellow the root was before you dried it.

Store the best roots separately, and use them up quickly.

The yellower the root, the more potent it is as a liver strengthener.

You'll find the best yellow docks in dry, sandy soil, where the plant must fight to survive. Such roots are deeply colored—even bright orange—in the center.

Roots grown in watery meadows usually are grayish white. These can be useful astringents, but because the world is full of astringent herbs, I see no need to dig such roots for that purpose.

The more flower stalks a dock has, the larger its taproot. I've dug roots as thick as 2 inches (5 cm), and as long as 18 inches (30–40 cm), but I've also dug yellow dock the size of a baby carrot.

EFFECTS AND USES

Yellow dock root is good for treating allergies and to strengthen the liver. It's appropriate for those with normal or low blood pressure, occasional digestive troubles (dairy and gluten intolerance don't count), and who have dry skin at least during the dry season (winter, in the north).

Yellow dock root is the wrong herb for those who work with solvents, who have high blood pressure, or who have had hepatitis. (Better for them are dandelion or burdock root.)

Use yellow dock to treat itchy hemorrhoids. Although laxative in larger doses, it's a stimulating one—one of the mildest such, but still it irritates the intestines to push food through faster. Instead, find out why you're constipated—food sensitivity? too little water? not enough exercise or dietary fiber?—and do something about that. If you must use a laxative, bulk ones such as flax or psyllium seed with sufficient water work more gently.

Yellow dock is good for coughs with an itchy throat. It moistens the mucous membranes, the itch stops, and then so does the cough.

Because yellow dock helps the liver and moistens mucous membranes, it's a good choice to treat allergic skin problems.

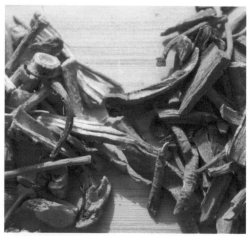

Dock roots dried in a dehydrator (left) and on an old bed sheet (right).

The taste is nothing to write home about, although it appeals to some people.

Rather than tincture the root, I usually mix it with tastier herbs to make a tea.

Decoction of yellow dock root

1–2 teaspoons dried sliced yellow dock root
nettles, thyme, mallow, or similar, to taste (optional)
1 cup (250 ml) cold water

Add the herb and water to a pan, bring to a boil, simmer 10 minutes, strain.

Drink one to three cups a day—more if the root was light yellow, less if it was dark yellow; more if you want a laxative effect; less if you're after other yellow dock effects.

Yellow dock tincture

From fresh root:

4 ounces (100 g) fresh roots in 1/6-inch (5 mm) slices, sticks, or bits
8 fluid ounces (1 cup, 200 ml) 190 proof grain alcohol (95 %)

From dried root:

4 ounces (100 g) dried roots in 1/6-inch (5 mm) slices, sticks, or bits
20 fluid ounces (500 ml) 100 proof grain alcohol (50 %)

Put the roots into a glass jar, cover with the alcohol, and close the lid tightly. Let steep for two to four weeks. Strain, bottle, and label (example: "Yellow dock, 1:5 50 %, 04.2021, Grandma's garden"). Dosage is 30–75 drops, one to three times a day.

Again—its color indicates its strength: the deeper the yellow, the more a root's active constituents, and so the smaller the needed dose.

FOOD USES

The ripe seeds of docks can be dried and mixed into flour.

Tart young dock leaves have a flavor like sorrel and can be added to salads.

The green parts contain oxalic acid, so use them with calcium-rich foods such as sunflower seeds or dairy.

WARNINGS

Don't use yellow dock as a laxative if you're pregnant. An irritated gut can stimulate womb cramping.

The leaves can trigger oxalic acid dermatitis in those with delicate skin.

Don't overdo it: too much yellow dock can cause kidney or bladder stones.

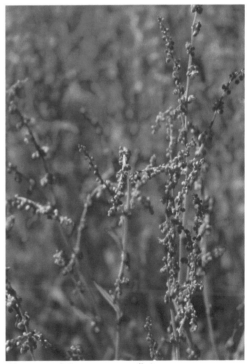

*Sheepsorrel (*Rumex acetosella*).*

SCIATICA

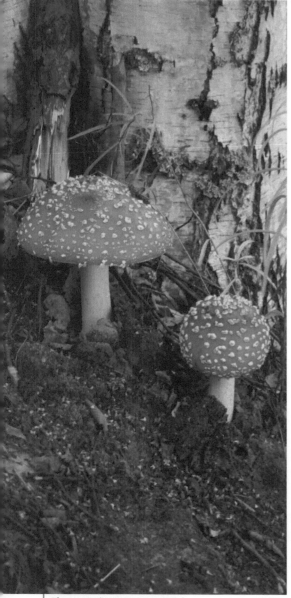

There is in fact a good old Finnish remedy for sciatica: a tincture of fly agaric or fly Amanita (*Amanita muscaria*)—applied externally, of course. Internal use can be rather fatal.

Make your tincture like this: cut one or two fly agarics (smaller than 4 inches or 10 cm) a bit above ground level into 1-inch (2–3 cm) dice, add them to a pint (500 ml) jar, cover with 80-proof vodka (38–40 percent alcohol), and steep for two or three weeks.

Decant through a sieve (don't press!), and then pour the stinky, grayish-pink liquid into a glass bottle. Label (example: "Poison! (skull picture), Fly agaric, September 2021"), and cap tightly.

When sciatica strikes, rub one to three drops of the tincture on the spine where the pain starts. The pain almost always stops immediately.

I got this recipe years ago from an elderly lady who attended one of my lectures, and I've remembered to tell it onward every time sciatica comes up. The response has followed this pattern: "Remember when you told us about fly agaric? We laughed, but when the fungus came up we decided to make the tincture after all. It's wonderful! The bottle has been passed all over our village!"

Always listen to elderly ladies.

And remember: fly agaric used internally is toxic!

Fly agaric (Amanita muscaria).

Index

144

146

Printed in the USA
CPSIA information can be obtained
at www.ICGtesting.com
JSHW042108181024
E13769200001B/2